ALSO BY JOHN SCHORK

A Journey of Honor

A Light in the Jungle

An Echo of War

Destiny in the Pacific

The Deadly Sky

The Falkenberg Riddle

The Flames of Deliverance

The King's Commander

The Right War

The Winds of Battle - Journey of James Addington

THE *LIGHT OF VICTORY*

John Schork

Cover composite derivation of Frank Hurley's WWI photo of infantry wounded near Zonnebeke Railway Station the morning after the first battle of Passchendaele, October 12, 1917.

Special thanks to Wikipedia, The National Library of Australia and The Frank Hurley Collection.

Cover and interior designs by Bill Glenn (JupiterPixel.com)

18380 SE Lakeside Dr.

Jupiter, FL 33469 USA

Printed in the United States of America

Wiki-tag:{{PD-US-expired} without restrictions}

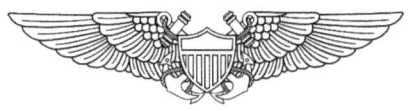

DEDICATED TO

Captain Dave Williams, USN

———— ·✛· ————

US Naval Academy Class of 1962
Commanding Officer Attack Squadron 145
Commanding Officer Attack Squadron 128
Commanding Officer Naval Air Station Whidbey Island

Counter-Attack

By Siegfried Sassoon - 1918

We'd gained our first objective hours before
While dawn broke like a face with blinking eyes,
Pallid, unshaven and thirsty, blind with smoke.
Things seemed all right at first. We held their line,
With bombers posted, Lewis guns well placed,
And clink of shovels deepening the shallow trench.
The place was rotten with dead; green clumsy legs
High-booted, sprawled and grovelled along the saps
And trunks, face downward, in the sucking mud,
Wallowed like trodden sand-bags loosely filled;
And naked sodden buttocks, mats of hair,
Bulged, clotted heads slept in the plastering slime.
And then the rain began, the jolly old rain !

A yawning soldier knelt against the bank,
Staring across the morning blear with fog;
He wondered when the Allemands would get busy;
And then, of course, they started with five-nines
Traversing, sure as fate, and never a dud.
Mute in the clamour of shells he watched them burst
Spouting dark earth and wire with gusts from hell,
While posturing giants dissolved in drifts of smoke.
He crouched and flinched, dizzy with galloping fear,
Sick for escape, loathing the strangled horror
And butchered, frantic gestures of the dead.

An officer came blundering down the trench:
"Stand-to and man the fire step !" On he went...
Gasping and bawling, "Fire-step...counter-attack !"
Then the haze lifted. Bombing on the right
Down the old sap: machine-guns on the left;
And stumbling figures looming out in front.
"O Christ, they're coming at us !" Bullets spat,
And he remembered his rifle... rapid fire...
And started blazing wildly... then a bang
Crumpled and spun him sideways, knocked him out
To grunt and wriggle: none heeded him; he choked
And fought the flapping veils of smothering gloom,
Lost in a blurred confusion of yells and groans...
Down, and down, and down, he sank and drowned,
Bleeding to death. The counter-attack had failed.

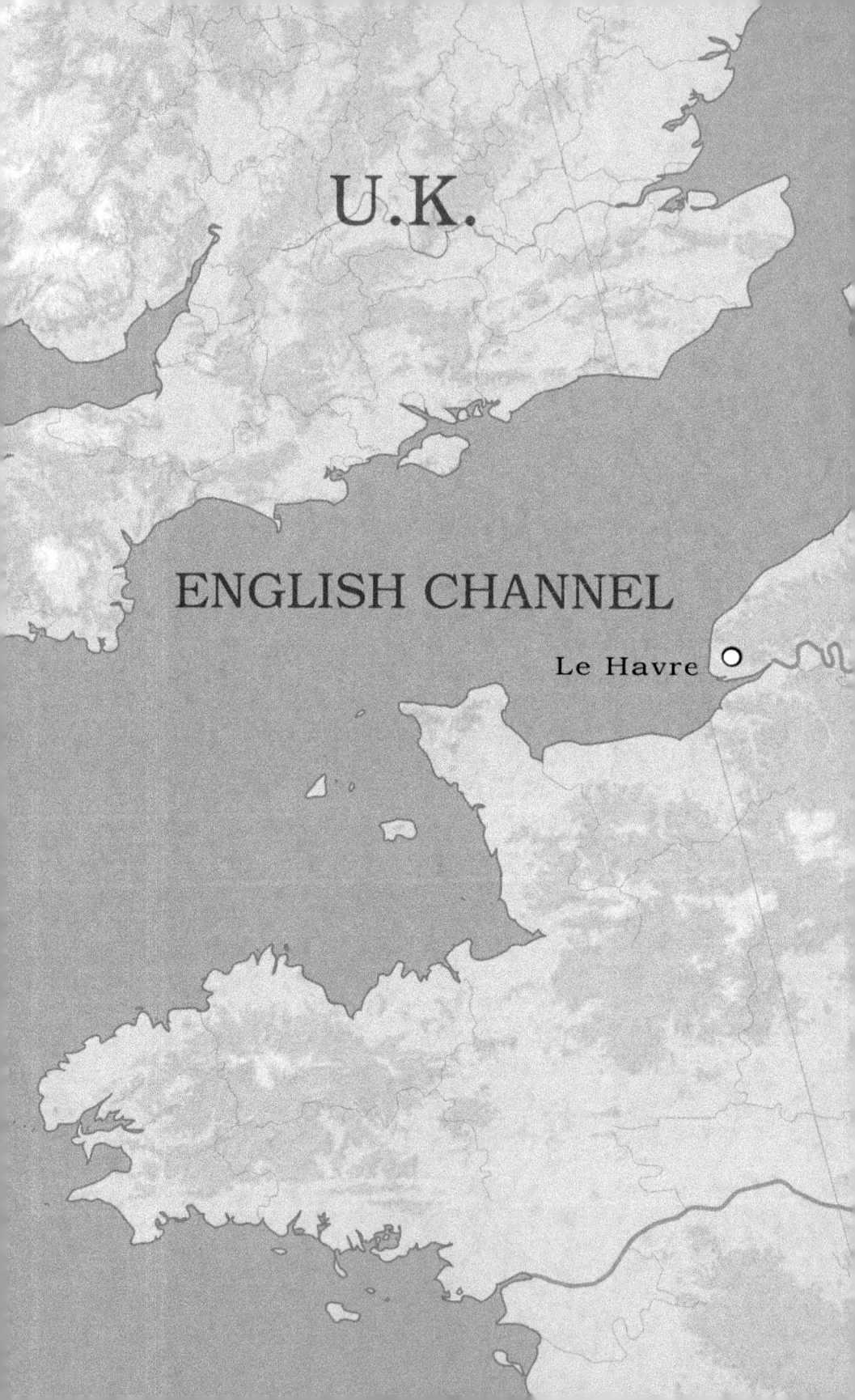

U.K.

ENGLISH CHANNEL

Le Havre

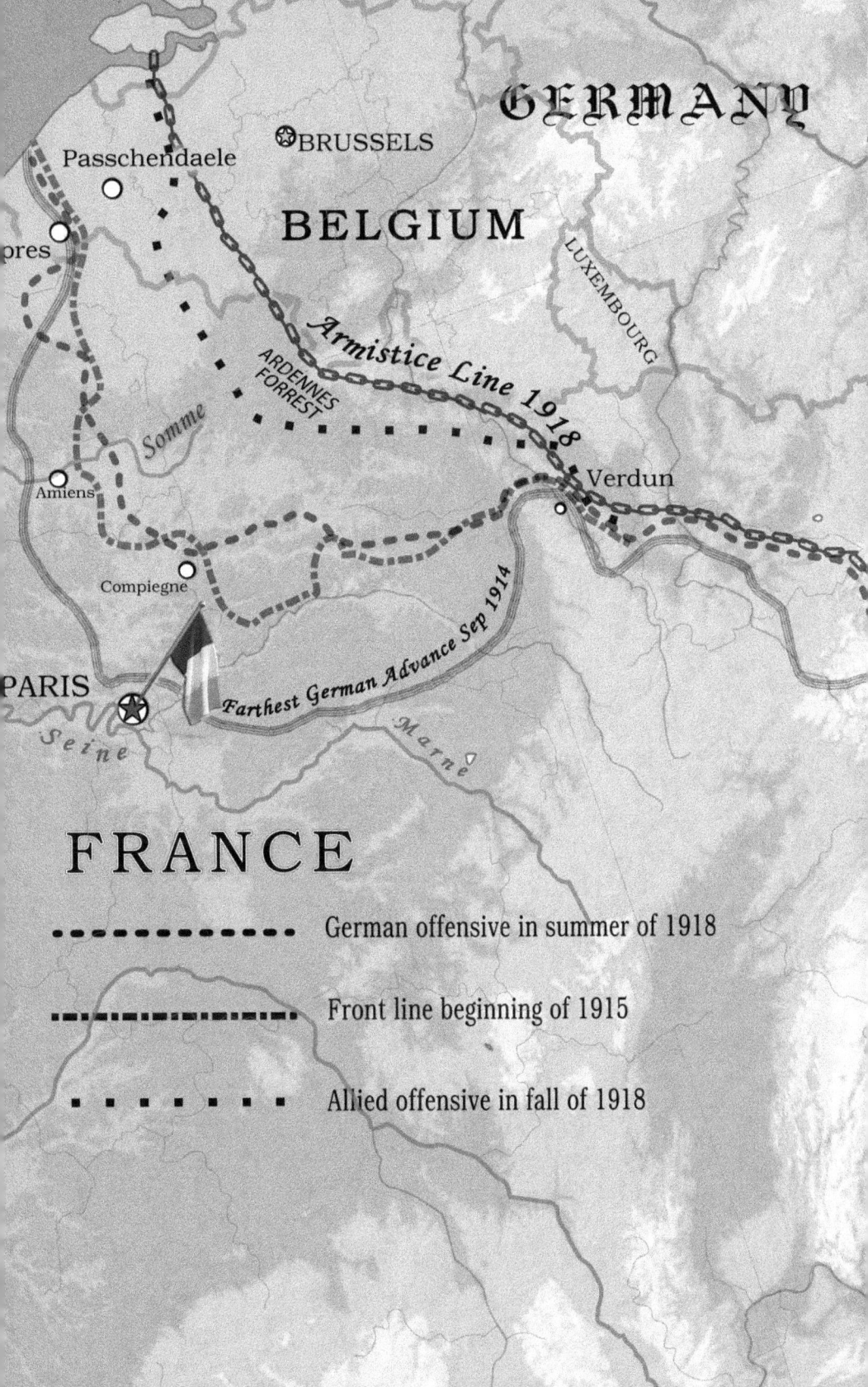

GERMANY

⊛BRUSSELS

BELGIUM

LUXEMBOURG

Passchendaele

pres

Armistice Line 1918

ARDENNES
FORREST

Somme

Verdun

Amiens

Compiegne

Farthest German Advance Sep 1914

PARIS

Seine

Marne

FRANCE

German offensive in summer of 1918

Front line beginning of 1915

Allied offensive in fall of 1918

Commonwealth War Casualties list 300,000 men of British and Commonwealth forces that remain classified as "missing" on the Western Front. Their bodies were never recovered. This does not include the 189,000 men buried but not identified and thus classified as "Unknown."

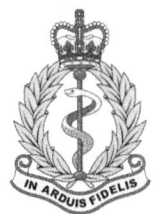

Prologue

Glasgow, Scotland U.K.
4 February 1949

During the years I spent in France from 1914 to 1918, we simply called the conflict which engulfed our lives, "the war" or some would call it "The Great War." In what must have been a desperate wish, H.G. Wells coined the phrase "the war that will end war." At some point that became popular as "the war to end all wars." But in 1939, as the horror of another world wide war descended on mankind, our time in France became The First World War. Despite the millions of lives lost on the battlefields around the world, mankind slid into what would become a more evil and tragic event for the nations and people of the world. At the time, the feeling of helplessness replicated the same emotions we felt in the summer of 1914 as nations stumbled into a conflict which quickly became The Second World War. The simplicity of the name reinforcing the terrible reality.

I rushed to the front as a young, incredibly young, doctor fresh from training, certain I would save lives and work miracles for the men of the British Army. Four years of war dispelled all thoughts of the noble physician toiling in the midst of shot and shell, bringing the lads home alive. Instead I saw men killed, wounded, gassed, shot, bayoneted, machine gunned, incinerated, frozen, buried alive, executed or simply vanish. An entire generation of young men on the battlefields and civilians of all ages sacrificed to the curse of mankind, war.

Now I sit in Glasgow, once more out of uniform. This last go-around, I returned to the Army as a surgeon stationed at the Royal Herbert Military

Hospital, Woolwich. Our job was to try and restore/rebuild the broken bodies from North Africa, then Europe. While a new war with a world of new drugs and procedures, it was very much like the first war. Young men fighting to return to a normal life with a future. I did not miss the sound of the guns, the rats, lice and brutal weather. But the daily struggle to heal the wounded was just as difficult. Truth be known, I could not have been anywhere else. Taking care of the lads was a duty I felt privileged to carry out. I always will.

Lieutenant Colonel David McFadden, DSC and Bar, MC

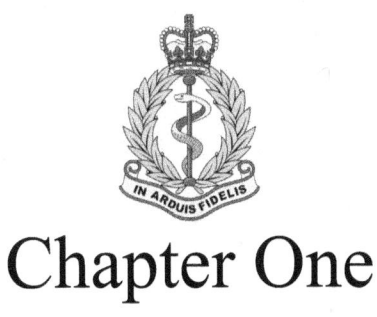

Chapter One

Into the Unknown

**Le Havre, France
3 September 1914**

Experience has taught me my expectations of a new location or experience invariably bear no resemblance to what I actually encounter. That lesson was never more on point as I arrived on the SS Mowbrey Canyon in Le Havre on a summer night in September of 1914. Wearing the uniform of a newly appointed lieutenant in the Royal Army Medical Corps, I watched the lights of the harbour as the ship slowly approached a long quay. Lit by a thin string of electrical lights on poles installed along the inboard side of the pier, I expected to arrive at a well-organized military assembly and distribution point. But that was simply my expectation.

From Portsmouth to Le Havre, a constant stream of commercial shipping had been conveying units of the newly constituted British Expeditionary Force as it attempted to build up enough forces to confront the wave of German divisions crashing though neutral Belgium. Common sense should have told me the chaos of war does not contribute to anything well organized, certainly not a major assembly point. Le Havre was no exception.

Walking down the brow, I found a maelstrom of people, animals, and equipment spread across the landing area, accompanied by much yelling, braying of animals, and the occasional whistle. It was quite discouraging.

Having left my baggage at the top of the ship's brow, I tried to locate anyone who might have some authority. After approaching several British non-commissioned officers, I came to the conclusion I needed to find the Railway Transport Officer, or RTO to find out what I might do to execute my written orders.

In my valise, I carried written orders from the Adjutant of the Highland Light Infantry to proceed to the headquarters in the field of the 2nd battalion of the regiment and present myself for active service. In my inexperience I was sure that once I found said RTO, I would immediately be recognized as a most important medical officer and given priority transportation to meet my regiment in the field. But as I said, expectations seldom play out as expected.

I say my regiment not only because I was ordered to report, but fifteen years before my father had seen service with the same regiment during the Boer conflict. My connection to the HLI went back many years.

As I walked through the throngs of troops, horses and equipment being offloaded from three streamers at the pier, I realized the magnitude of what was happening in this area of the French port.

If fact, it took me an hour to find the tent which housed the rail transport section and the RTO.

"Over there, lieutenant," a harried sergeant told me, pointing to a major at a far desk,

I approached the RTO, who held his head in both hands, staring down at an open notebook on his desk.

Not sure exactly what to do, I came to attention and saluted.

"Lieutenant McFadden, reporting to the Highland Light Infantry, sir."

For a moment the officer did nothing, then slowly raised his head.

"What?"

"McFadden, sir. Highland Light Infantry."

"And exactly what do you expect me to do about that, Mr. McFadden of the Highland Light Infantry?"

I noticed the major's collar was completely unfastened and he badly needed a shave.

"I'm not quite sure, sir. I was told I should find you. I assume to arrange transportation to my regiment."

The major rubbed his face as he sat back in the chair.

"Christ," he muttered.

"Sir?"

He looked at me with what I took as disdain.

"You may not know this, lieutenant. But the Highland Light Infantry is part of Second Corps. At this moment, Second Corps is falling back to the southwest from the border of Belgium in the general direction of Paris. I have no bloody idea where they are or where they're going to be. You'd be well advised to stay here until the situation stabilizes. Now get out, I have work to do."

I started to salute, then saw he had returned to his paperwork. Turning, I walked out of the tent into the night.

When I left Glasgow, my father told me whatever I encountered, I should "do my duty." Certainly, in the last four years of my surgical residency in London I did what was required and even more. But here, what is my duty? It seemed straightforward to me, find my regiment and take care of the wounded.

Sounds of an altercation came from down a row between the storage tents. I stopped, turned my head and was bowled over by a body falling sideways. The two of us went down onto the graveled path as another man ran by into the darkness.

Getting to my hand and knees, I saw the other man lay on his back, hand to his left side.

"Blimey, the bawbag nicked me."

Looking closer I saw the uniform of a British private missing only his hat.

"Here soldier, let me help you up."

Pulling him to his feet I saw his right hand was covered in blood. Looking around I saw a bench along one side of the nearest tent.

"Sit over here."

The man sat down, the bloody hand to his side.

"Criminy, it hurts," he said, wincing with the pain.

"I'm a doctor, let me see that."

He unbuttoned his jacket and by the light of the nearest electric light, I saw a slashing wound across the man's ribs. My experience in London included a number of street fights and luckily the ribs often provide sufficient protection to prevent grievous wounds. A quick exam confirmed my initial opinion. Pulling out a clean handkerchief from my tunic, I folded it four times and pressed it against the wound.

"Here, press hard, the bleeding should stop."

We sat for a moment, then I asked, "What was that all about?"

The man hesitated then said, "Noh much," sounding evasive.

"I see, just an argument."

"Right."

"Are you with these troops that just landed?"

"Uh, no . . . sir."

He apparently decided some amount of military decorum was called for. I suspect he was not used to the military. My indoctrination at the Royal Army Medical College in Millbank had given me just enough information to ask appropriate questions.

"What is you unit?"

"The 531st Motor Transport Company, sir."

"And where would they be?"

"I honestly dunno. When I left four days ago, they were near Soissons, just south of the Aisne river. Everyone's pulling back. They could be anywhere."

"How did you get to Le Havre?"

"On me motorcycle, I'm a dispatch rider."

"What's your name?"

"Jones, sir. Private Jones."

"And do you have a first name, Private Jones?"

"Ryan, but I'm called Jonesy."

Well, Private Jones, let's go back to my ship. I have supplies there and we'll get that wound of yours bandaged up properly."

Private Ryan Jones, if that was really his name, was a tall young man, probably six feet three inches, but spare, weighing maybe twelve stone. He seemed a likeable sort, telling me he'd been in France for the past month. The first major encounter between the BEF and the German's had taken place near the Belgium town of Mons on the 23rd of August and the BEF had been pulling back ever since.

"There you go," I said as I finished bandaging his side.

"Thanks, doc."

"You're a dispatch rider. Did you bring dispatches to Le Havre?"

"No, three bags of post for home."

"How could you carry three mail bags on a motorcycle?"

"Too easy, I 'ave a sidecar."

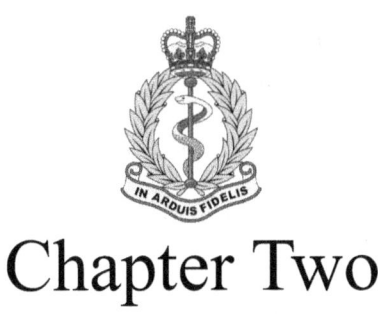

Chapter Two

To the Front

The Le Havre Tancarville Road
4 September 1914

At first light, we departed the port area heading west in the direction of Compiegne. While rumors were rampant across the holding area, examination of a map Jonesy had with him put Compiegne in the path the RTO had described. In addition, my stalwart driver heard the name mentioned by a lieutenant just before he left the front. Our destination was, at least, an educated guess.

In the early hours of the morning, I learned Private Jones was a most ingenious individual. By the time the sun rose, I was equipped with a set of goggles, suitable for the passenger in his Triumph Roadster's sidecar. My driver looked much more the soldier in the light of day, with a Webley revolver on his hip, a large pair of leather gauntlets and a leather outer jacket

After leaving most of my extraneous belongings with the first mate of the Mowbrey Canyon, Jonesy located a duffle bag for my basic uniform items and a medical bag I put together prior to leaving London.

Confidant he knew his way, I was able to observe the traffic of war as we left the built-up area of the city. Though dominated by horse drawn wagons, a number of trucks were in evidence heading to the front. It was interesting the trucks were all French, along with the occasional small sedan. It struck me I did not see any motor vehicles being offloaded from our steamers in the port. I knew the majority of the logistical support for the troops was horse drawn, but I was led to believe motor driven ambulances were available for the wounded. Perhaps they were all at the front.

The summer heat left the road hard and dusty, the paved portion of the road having ended shortly after leaving the city. Jonesy told me about half of our troops were able to entrain for the front, however, many were required to march, a grueling effort in the summer heat. In short order, I found my young driver was rather adept at avoiding potholes, trucks and the plodding horse drawn wagons. He seemed to enjoy the speed available to him, often opening the throttle when the opportunity presented itself. I must admit I found this rather exhilarating, having little experience with any type of motor vehicle. Any traveling I had done during my years at school in Edinburgh had been by rail. Once in residency in London, there was seldom time to leave the hospital other than to return to my lodgings for a bath and change of clothes.

My last four years, which culminated with my final exam for membership in the Royal College of Surgeons, had but one purpose, to learn the art and science of surgery. In order to accomplish this, there was no time for anything other than study and practical application. I was most fortunate to have studied directly under Sir William Cheyne, the chief of surgery at King's College Hospital and one of the most renowned surgeons in England. While a hard taskmaster, I am confident no one ever had a better course of instruction. I am also sure what I encounter on the battlefield will make me a better surgeon and doctor.

Within an hour, I truly felt like my body was covered by the dust of the road. The temperature rose along with the sun and sweat combined with the dust to form a clinging paste to my face. The initial thrill of the ride soon became a tedious jolting, accompanied by the whine of the Roadster's engine. But we were advancing in what I believed was the right direction.

"Let's pull over up ahead," I yelled at Jonesy.

He nodded.

At a large clearing, he wheeled the bike well clear of traffic, over to the edge of a field under cultivation. The quiet when he shut the engine down was startling.

"Right, there we go," he said, pulling off his goggles and helmet.

I reached for my handkerchief to wipe my face and remembered it laying on the floor of the first mate's stateroom on the ship. Lesson learned, carry extra handkerchiefs.

"Where are we?" I asked.

He reached down to a saddlebag on the left side of the gas tank. Pulling out the map, he spread it over the tank, handing one side to me.

"We've gone 'bout fifteen miles, so I think we're here. Makes it fifteen miles to Lillibonne, and there's a Service Corps depot. We can get petrol and likely some eats."

I realized I hadn't eaten anything in my haste to get on the road and my stomach was grumbling. Lesson two, try to carry something to eat if possible.

"Here," Jonesy said and handed me a canteen,

The water was warm, but welcome and I decided carrying a canteen also made sense. I was rapidly figuring out that in a war zone, one should plan on being self-sufficient as it seems nothing is readily available.

"If you're hungry, I've got bully beef, but we can get better at the depot."

I nodded, the voice of experience was speaking. The sound of heavy equipment came from behind us. Turning I saw a large French truck towing a massive artillery piece. My God, the gun was twenty feet long, with huge wheels. As the truck went by, I saw there were two more of the large guns following under tow. The reality of the war came crashing home. These guns were on their way to fire at the German army. Until now it hadn't seemed there was a real war occurring. And now it was apparent, the conflict was not far away. I couldn't help but wonder, what would I find? I had no idea, and my expectations did not even have a frame of reference. The few pictures I had seen in the London papers were generally of groups of soldiers standing around equipment. But time would tell, most certainly.

The depot in Lillebonne consisted of perhaps fifteen tents outside the town proper with a number of vehicles, wagons and horses parked and tethered. There was a lorry with a large container for petrol under a group of trees.

"There's the petrol. They hide it under trees so the German airplanes can't see it. Makes a good target."

I involuntarily looked to the skies, which were clear of any flying craft.

"German airplanes?"

"You'll see them a lot. They're looking for targets. Sometimes you see our planes chasing 'em."

"Targets for what?" I asked.

"Artillery. The Hun artillery's damned good, I'll tell ya."

Again, the voice of experience.

"There's the dispatcher tent," Jonesy said, pointing to a large square tent with a sign that said, "Check In Here."

"Why don't you see if they know anything about your outfit."

"Can't you do that?" I asked.

"Well, better I don't. They'll send me off to Timbuktu and you'd be stranded."

His logic made sense, but I also wondered if there was more to it?

Entering the tent, I saw three men sitting at a table covered with a very large map. The senior man was a major, so I approached the table and saluted.

"Hello, I'm Doctor McFadden, enroute to the Highland Light Infantry."

The three men looked up from the map, and the major actually smiled.

"Suspect they'll be needing doctors in a big way. Let me check the latest updates."

He flipped through a pile of flimsy papers.

"Here you go. Looks like they're moving toward Compiegne. This was as of last night, so rather hard to pin down. It looks like the army is trying to set up a defensive line protecting Paris, but no one knows where that will be. From what we hear, whether you find them or not, there is plenty of need for medical officers everywhere on the line."

I pulled out our map and made several marks to remind me what he said.

"Thank you, sir. I'll be on my way."

"Do you have transport, doctor."

"Oh yes, I do indeed," I said, easing out of the tent. "Thanks, very much."

Seeing Jonesy standing by a tree, I walked over.

"Compiegne."

"Right then. Let's get some food, then on our way."

The mess tent had a serving area at one end and four tables with chairs. A few men were eating as we entered and picked up tin plates and cups. The fare was simple, boiled potatoes and a bully beef gravy. Thank heavens, there was a plentiful supply of very decent tea.

Satiated, we resumed our journey, the early afternoon sun driving the temperature into a slightly uncomfortable range. The breeze from our motorcycle was very much appreciated. Our study of the map dictated our next destination would be Rouen, which was approximately one hundred road miles from Compiegne.

Making good time, we entered Rouen in midafternoon. A large military presence was evident as we passed through the center of the city, paralleling the river Seine for several miles. Jonesy knew a transportation depot was located in Beauvais, which we could reach by sundown. A chance to refuel, get some food and rest sounded attractive as my body was beginning to rebel at the constant pounding of the motorcycle.

After several wrong turns, we arrived at the service depot as twilight began to deepen the shadows of the day. I was surprised at not only the size of the depot, but the number of vehicles, both motor and horse drawn parked across a large field. Two wooden open sided barns on one side of the field were the only permanent structures. At least twenty large tents ringed the field with soldiers milling around what turned out to be the messing facility. Cooking fires on the backside of the large tent confirmed the cooks were hard at work on the evening meal.

Jonesy again found a relatively inconspicuous spot to park the motorcycle which also offered a sturdy fencepost to secure the locking chain. I searched out the operations tent to see if there might be any update on the Highland Light Infantry's location.

"Compiegne? If you're going there, you better be able to speak German," a very fat major said in reply to my inquiry. While the man smelled of liquor, he seemed to have a good feel for what was happening across the French countryside. He pointed to a map.

"I'd recommend heading to Meaux. Our chaps are setting up a defensive line here, between the French 5th and 6th armies, about 50 miles southeast from here. How are you traveling?"

I paused then said, "Motorcycle."

"Ah, no problem, the roads are decent."

Taking a second look at my uniform, the major asked, "Are you a doctor?"

"Yes, I am."

"We have a load of wounded come in earlier today. No orders, and the field hospitals are all on the move. Not sure what we're supposed to do with them, but perhaps you could take a look?"

"Of course, where are these men?"

Jonesy and I found a large, covered wagon under a large tree. A small cooking fire burned near the rear of the wagon and two men sat next to the fire.

"Are there wounded men here?" I asked as we walked up.

The two men looked up.

"In the wagon," one of the men said, turning back to the fire.

"What unit," I asked, falling back on my minimal military training.

"The Fusiliers," the man said.

I was not totally unaware of the military world and said, "Be more specific."

He looked back surprised and got up.

"The Royal Scot Fusiliers, sir."

"And you are?"

"Corporal Rosyth."

"I'm Doctor McFadden, here to examine the wounded. Are you a medical orderly?"

"Just a corporal."

"What were your orders?"

The man shrugged. "I got wounded, and the captain told me to take them men behind the lines. Course no one told me where to go, so been trying to find a hospital."

I noticed by the light of the fire, a dirty bandage wrapped Corporal Rosyth's lower left leg.

"Right. Let's take a look at what we've got."

Jonesy followed me with my bag.

Climbing into the wagon, the smell hit me immediately. Urine, feces, and rotting straw. The interior was dimly lit by a lantern.

There were nine stretchers in the wagon. The men lay uncovered, their dark uniforms broken by bandages evident on each. One man at the front of the wagon moaned quietly and rocked back and forth. The rest of the wounded were quiet and still.

"Ryan, get me clean drinking water and see if those men have any medical supplies with them."

"Aye."

I decided to make a quick survey of the men to see if there were any critical emergencies I should deal with first.

As I moved to the first man I wondered if this was the normal state our wounded found themselves.

Looking down I saw eyes that were open as was the mouth. My immediate reaction was the man was clearly dead. The lack of a pulse and cool skin confirmed my diagnosis. He had a large blood-soaked bandage around his right thigh. Blood also covered his lower leg and the straw under him. Christ, the man bled to death.

Multiple wounds on the next man must have come from a shell burst. A dozen unbandaged holes in his tunic surrounded a large bandage covering his shoulder. The man opened his eyes when I put my hand on his brow.

"Hello soldier, I'm Doctor McFadden, what's your name?"

The man said, "Thompson," in a weak voice.

"I'm going to examine your shoulder. Just lay still."

A jagged wound ran across his chest, blood still oozing through the congealed scab and dirt.

"When were you wounded, son?"

"Two days ago…I think."

My survey revealed one other man dead, the remainder were in various states of shock, dehydrated and most were feverish. Over the next three hours, Jonesy and I replaced all of the bloody bandages. Thank God there was iodine in the medical bag and I was able to do a reasonable job of cleaning the many wounds. We also administered water, which the men desperately needed. For pain I had aspirin and a bottle of codeine pills in my bag. The lack of morphine was a situation I vowed to never be in again. My personal preparations had been sorely lacking for a doctor proceeding into a combat area. But now I knew.

Corporal Rosyth made a broth from canned beef for the men who could take nourishment. We fed them the broth and it seemed to pick up several of the wounded noticeably.

Jonesy and I were finishing up in the wagon when we heard a cry outside. Emerging from the wagon I saw Corporal Rosyth laying on the ground next to the fire, his mate kneeling next him.

Rolling the corporal on his back, I saw he was conscious but not coherent, muttering something I couldn't understand. He was running a fever, sweat covered his face and his pulse was rapid.

"You, what's your name?"

"Freeman, sir, Private Freeman."

"Go get a blanket."

Jonesy and I did a quick examination of Rosyth and determined his leg wound was the only major issue. I suspect he also had been treated simply by binding the wound on his lower leg, which was clearly a gunshot. I knew some physicians, particularly in France, advocated taking no action at the front except binding wounds, then sending the men to the rear. It appears that some of my British colleagues must feel the same way.

"Here's the blanket, doctor."

"Good, now go get the lantern."

Under the light of a lantern, Jonesy and I laid the corporal on a blanket. Cutting off his trouser leg, I used a diluted solution of iodine to thoroughly clean his leg, paying particular attention to the entry wound. There was no exit wound making me think this wound might have been a bullet glancing off something else. While I did have two scalpels, I only had one clamp. The chances of needing a clamp were minimal, but one never could be sure. It was one more example of the need to be prepared better. With no type of anesthetic, I was prepared to use some of my Glenfiddich, which was carefully wrapped in several of my shirts in the duffel bag. As it turned out, the corporal procured a bottle of brandy during his trip from the front. We had him drink one glass, which was the equivalent of about six ounces. Giving him thirty minutes for the liquor to take effect, I started by gently probing the wound. The bullet path had missed the bone, traversing the fleshy part of the calve. It appeared to me the path was straight, and I encountered what felt like the bullet. As I evaluated the problem, it struck me the least invasive operation would be to simply access the bullet from the other side of the calve where it likely would have exited. Gently pushing, it felt like the bullet was actually close to the surface.

"Ryan, hand me the iodine bottle."

I thoroughly cleaned the area intended for the incision.

"You gonna cut him there?" Jonesy asked.

"I am, and if I'm right, the bullet should be right under the skin."

"Criminey," he said with some degree of awe.

An incision, careful insertion of my forceps and out came a partially deformed bullet. It appeared the projectile had indeed hit something prior to lodging in Corporal Rosyth's lower leg.

"He's good as new." Jonesy said.

"Unless some of his trouser leg was pulled into the wound."

The young man looked confused, so I continued.

"Any foreign matter can lead to infection. Often a bullet will pull clothing into the wound and can cause big problems. So, we search for anything that which could contaminate the wound."

"I see."

After further examination I did find a piece of fabric which I was able to extract. Jonesy appeared to have a revelation as he examined the piece of cloth from the corporal's leg.

"So, he'll be all right?"

I nodded.

"Never any guarantees, but all things being equal he should make a normal recovery."

"He needs a bandage. Would you like to learn how to do it?"

"Could I?"

"Certainly, hand me that gauze roll from the bag."

Ten minutes later, my dispatch rider made his first foray into the world of patient care.

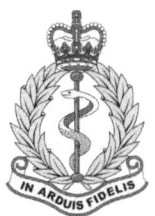

Chapter Three

"My God, we have a prodigy among us."

Beauvais Transport Depot
5 September 1914

Leaving the wagonload of wounded in the care of Private Freeman, we left for Meaux. The private was ordered to go directly to the hospital at Rouen. I felt certain the hospital would take the men as patients with the large military presence in the town. If he was refused, he was to go immediately to the Rouen Depot and find a senior officer.

Within an hour, the evidence of a massive military buildup was everywhere. Checkpoint and traffic directing sections were present along with more and more military units. It was clear the area we were traversing was allocated to the French army. After being stopped several times, we understood these were units of the French Sixth Army, taking up defensive positions. The military police or gendarmerie continued directing us to the southeast where they understood the British Expeditionary Force was also taking up defensive positions. In addition, they warned us the Germans were moving rapidly south and to be very careful lest we blunder into enemy forces.

On hearing of the German proximity, I took out my own Webley revolver and made sure it was loaded. While medical personnel were supposedly non-combatants, the stories of German brutality told me to err on the side of safety.

At midday, we saw our first British troops. They were in a column under arms, marching along a wide dirt road, moving east. Several mounted officers could be seen, obviously in command of the group. I pointed out an officer riding up the left side of the column and directed Jonesy to pull up alongside of him.

The horse reacted to the sound of the motorcycle, but the rider had him well under control. I exited the sidecar and approached the rider who I could now see was a lieutenant colonel. Sitting upright in the saddle, he looked the very epitome of the British officer. He looked young for a lieutenant colonel, very athletic if my guess was right. Other than a mustache, he looked rather plain, but still impressive.

I saluted and said, "Sir, My name is McFadden, I'm looking for the Highland Light Infantry. Might you have some idea where I could find them."

He grinned at me and said, "Look no further, lieutenant. This is the second battalion of the Lights. I'm Abernathy."

Our search appeared to be over.

"Shall we fall in the column, sir?"

"Actually, you can help us. We're marching to join the first battalion of the Scots. They're supposedly holding positions on this road further east, along with our supply and medical staffs. If you can move east, find them and let me know where exactly they are, I would be most appreciative."

"Yes, sir."

"You said your name was McFadden?"

"Yes, sir."

Four miles down the road we encountered a large number of troops deployed across a wide field. Wagons, horses and one truck were parked by a tent with a flag on a ten-foot pole near the entrance. In short order we confirmed this was not only the first battalion of the Royal Scots, but also their regimental headquarters.

"Ryan, go back and let Lieutenant Colonel Abernathy know we found the Royal Scots. I'm going to try and find our medical staff."

Twenty minutes of wandering around the encampment led me to a copse of trees with a large number of wooden crates arranged in a semi-circle. Men in their shirt sleeves were unpacking the crates while another was putting up a canvas tent.

"I'm looking for the Highland Light Infantry medical officer."

A skinny man, put down a canvas bag he was pulling from a crate and looked at me. He pulled a handkerchief from his pocket and wiped his face.

"Oh, lieutenant, right, he should be over in that direction, by the big table."

"Major Ashcroft?"

"Yes, sir, that's him."

My father told me Ashcroft, a career army man, held the position for the battalion. He didn't know much about the man, but assumed he knew his job, or he wouldn't have been appointed to the job.

"What's your name, soldier?"

"Musgrave, Corporal Musgrave, sir. Medical orderly."

"Nice to meet you corporal. What's going on here?"

"Setting up our dressing station. We've been moving for the last two days and now we're going to dig in."

The entire area looked like complete chaos, but I assumed everyone knew their jobs.

"Please carry on, Corporal Musgrave."

I found the table and saw a well-turned-out major standing beside it. Of medium height, his short, cropped hair was just visible under his cap.

Saluting, I said, "Major Ashcroft?"

The man turned, slightly surprised, returned the salute and said, "I am. What may I do to help you, lieutenant?

"David McFadden, sir, reporting for duty."

"Ah, we've been expecting you. Actually, I thought you would have found us earlier."

"Yes, sir, of course."

"I understand you have been at King's College in London?"

"The last four years, actually."

"Four years, you say?"

"Studying surgery."

Ashcroft turned to look at David.

"Surgery, really. And how far did you get in the course?"

"I passed my College of Surgeon's exam in February."

"The RMCS exam?"

"Yes, sir. I was studying under Doctor Cheyne and he stood for me to take the exam."

"After only four years?"

"Yes sir."

"My God, we have a prodigy among us."

I had no reply to the sarcastic comment from the major. Again, I fell back on my brief training.

"Orders, sir?"

"Find Sergeant Loefler, he'll take care of billeting. Once you've dropped your gear off, report back to me."

As I started my search for the sergeant, I saw Jonesy pull into the encampment and roll up to me.

"Message delivered. Colonel Abernathy seems a good enough sort. Nah like the officers at my camp."

The thought struck me, my assistant, as I had come to think of him, officially belonged to a motor transport company. He was now absent from his station and without authorization. For now, it would probably not be a problem with thousands of soldiers on the move. But at some point, he must go back to his unit.

Twenty minutes later I was being directed by Sergeant Loefler, the medical staff's leading non-commissioned officer, to an area where several large tarps had been erected. Jonesy followed, my duffel bag in hand. I carried my medical bag.

These were temporary officer's quarters, and I saw duffel bags, a few suitcases and bed rolls arranged in two rows under each tarp. Certainly, only the most basic protection, but it was what I would expect in a war zone.

In short order I selected a spot and was ready to leave when another officer ducked under the edge of the tarp. A rather slender man, he grinned at me under his mop of very red hair.

"Hello, there, just arriving?"

"Yes, in from Le Havre. David McFadden," I said, extending my hand.

"James Pomeroy," he answered. "Everyone calls me Jimmy."

"Well, Jimmy, it's nice to meet you. But I really do have to push on, Major Ashcroft is waiting for me."

"Ashcroft, the sawbones?"

I was taken aback. "Sawbones" was a term I had heard before, but I honestly did not care for it. I preferred the common shortened term of "doc," which seemed to be collegial as opposed to "sawbones" which was derogatory. In my opinion anyway.

"Yes, Doctor Ashcroft."

Jimmy took a closer look at my uniform and colored.

"Oh, I see. You're a doctor also."

I smiled but there wasn't much warmth in it.

"Yes, that's right. Now I really must go."

Walking across the field, I stopped and turned to Jonesy.

"Why don't you take a tour of the camp. I'm sure there are things we both should know, and I suspect I'll be busy with the senior medical officer.

"Right."

Major Ashcroft pointed out the general layout of the camp. He seemed slightly detached, but for a career army man I assumed he had seen all of this many times before.

"No idea how long we'll be here," he explained. "I'm told the French will attack soon, which might involve us. But you never know about these things."

Across the open area, I saw the battalion was arriving with Colonel Abernathy riding at its head.

"We are setting up a receiving station to be prepared for any casualties. Our job will be to do whatever we can and get the wounded on their way to Rouen."

"Rouen, sir?"

"Quite so. A major field hospital will be set up near the civilian hospital. From that point, they'll be moved to one of the channel ports for return to England."

"I encountered a wounded transport wagon on my way here. The wounded were in a disgraceful state, two had even died and no one noticed. How will we transport our wounded?"

"Really up to the quartermasters, you know. Not our business. Over the last month, they have used wagons when needed."

"We were told motorized ambulances had been landed in France and were available," I said.

"We had twenty motorized ambulances for the entire Second Corps. Ludicrous. I'll stick with horses all the time." He watched the marching troops wind their way into the center of the open field. "Now, with the troops arriving, it's important we provide sanitary guidance. I am appointing you the battalion latrine officer."

"Latrine officer?"

"Indeed. It is my experience both before the war and certainly since Belgium that the other ranks will squat and defecate wherever it pleases them. That is simply unacceptable. I want you to coordinate with each of the companies to find a good location and ensure the latrines are constructed according to army field regulations."

I thought to myself this is absurd, but I guess it's the way of the military. Until I'm more familiar with the rules of conduct all I can do is follow orders.

"Yes, sir, of course."

While I knew the primary purpose of the British Expeditionary Force was to defeat the Germans, I also became aware field latrines should normally be two feet wide and six feet long. They should have some type of privacy covers for the users. Periodically, lime or other disinfectants should be applied to reduce odors and insects. At some point, they should be filled in and relocated, always a good distance from any food preparation areas and ideally downwind from the prevailing wind direction.

Armed with that knowledge, I visited each of the four companies, found the first sergeant and expressed my interest in their facilities. I was greeted by varied reactions from exasperation to mirth. Trying to exhibit my most professional demeanor, I conducted the tour and returned to my tent to find Jonesy talking with an officer.

"You must be McFadden," the tall officer said, extending his hand. "James Edwards, a pleasure to meet you."

We shook hands and I noticed he wore the Royal Army Medical Corps insignia on the collar of his tunic. His sleeve insignia told me he was also a lieutenant.

"I've been waiting for your arrival. The battalion is allocated two doctors for the field. I am one and you, my friend, are the other one."

"It's all a bit overwhelming, you have some guidance for the new boy, I'm sure."

"We're both new, David. I've only been here for three weeks. Ashcroft was the only doctor for the first part of the campaign."

"He's assigned me as the latrine officer."

He smiled and said, "He's a career army type. A bit stiff if you ask me. He was recently promoted, and this billet calls for a captain. He feels he should be moving up the chain, more responsibility and all that. Rubbish, I say."

It seems I might have encountered a kindred spirit.

"Let's take a walk, he said."

"You were here for the battle around Mons?" I asked as we crossed the camp.

"I was. Only here for two weeks prior to that, so had to learn by doing."

"Many casualties?"

"Actually no. At the Battle of Mons as they are now calling it, most of the casualties were among the Royal Scots and the Gordon Highlanders. We moved south and never saw much action."

That helped me understand what was going on around me. They were all the same as I was, a novice to war. It seemed we would learn together.

"James, where are you from?"

"Just south of Cambridge, a small village called Harston."

"Married?" I asked.

"I am, Sally. And with have a two year old, Timothy, although I just call him Timmy."

"Are you going back to practice there after the war?"

"I think I'd like to. A small town where I know everyone is my cup of tea."

I wondered what I would do after the war. Joining my father's practice would certainly be expected. But the excitement of a big hospital in London is attractive. Perhaps by the time the war is over, I'll have a better idea.

The medical treatment area consisted of four large tents, with supply cases stacked up beside each tent. I saw many stretchers standing vertically against one stack of boxes. A strange contraption stood in the center of the tents. It appeared to be a large medal box that rested on a wagon bed. A pipe ran up from the box and I realized it was a chimney. The apparatus was some type of portable stove. Quite smart I thought.

In short order, James showed me the layout which included a supply tent, two examination tents and a procedure tent, where more complicated treatment was to take place.

"Surgery?"

"I wouldn't go so far as that. Ashworth has very definite ideas about the purpose of a battalion aid station. Bind the wound and get them on their way, he likes to say."

I relayed my encounter with the wagon full of casualties, how even simple procedures might have saved the lives of at least two of the soldiers.

"I don't know what the most important thing for him is, the need to keep the receiving station clear to accept new casualties or the lack of capacity for the wounded."

"It seems to me simple procedures don't compromise casualty evacuation. In fact, they help with the ultimate survival rate if we can reduce danger sooner rather than later."

James lit a cigarette, blew out the smoke and said, his tone much more serious than before, "Just be warned, Ashcroft is old school. Cross him and I don't see it going well for you."

We were silent walking back to the quartering area.

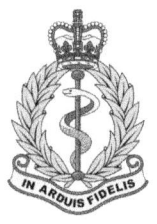

Chapter Four

"Our lads push off in two hours."

**British Encampment north of Meaux
6 September 1914**

Rest did not come that night, whether it was the new surroundings or my own excitement I didn't know. I was stiff and tired as rose and put on my shoes. Having slept in my uniform, minus tunic, I felt the war was already winning.

Jimmy Pomeroy stood over by a portable water bag. Several basin pans were stacked on a wood bench, and I filled one with cool water.

"Good morning, McFadden," Jimmy said as he wiped his face. "Another schilling from the King, eh?"

"Hello, Jimmy."

I quickly washed my face, shaved and brushed my teeth. I brought two tubes of Euthymol paste, not knowing how available it might be in the field. What I had not brought along was a towel, so a rather expensive handkerchief served the purpose. Perhaps Jonesy could find a towel. If I was able get a bath or shower, I was sure my handkerchief would not suffice.

Putting away my toiletries, I heard a rumbling to the west. There were clouds in the sky and as I looked to the darkened western horizon it seemed there were flashes highlighted against those clouds. In a moment I realized it was French artillery. This was war.

Was this the attack Ashcroft had mentioned? If the French attacked, we might be required to do the same. I needed to find Major Ashcroft and report.

"No, sir. I haven't seen the major this morning. Have you tried the mess?"

The duty sergeant pointed me across the camp to a large tent which he said was the officer's mess tent.

I found a dozen officers sitting at two tables, having their morning meal. Seeing James Edwards, I sat down next to him.

"Good morning," I said.

"Hello, David. Gentlemen, this is David McFadden our newest doctor."

Four officers sitting across the table smiled and acknowledged my presence as they continued to tuck into their breakfast.

"Nothing fancy, I'm afraid, but it will keep you alive."

As it turned out, the cooks were out of eggs, but did provide a quite suitable porridge. I was happy to be offered coffee or tea and I chose coffee, having become devoted to the harsh liquid during my four years at King's College.

After one cup of coffee, and a bowl of porridge, James walked with me to the medical area. Jonesy stood waiting for me at one of the examination tents, his uniform looking brushed and his face clean shaven. Perhaps he had the makings of a medical orderly in training.

Major Ashcroft called for a staff muster at 0800. In the intervening twenty minutes, James conducted a walk-through of the area, introducing me to staff that had not been there the previous afternoon. My impression was the personnel were efficient and well trained. It would be validated when the casualties began arriving.

"The French will be starting their advance this morning. Our lads will also push off in about two hours."

The group included James and the noncommissioned medical orderlies and assistants for the battalion.

Major Ashcroft had no map but would point to the north as he discussed his understanding of the attack plan. Our battalion would be leading the advance, and we would be prepared to deal with casualties within the immediate area. He went over several points which all seemed to be focused on rapid treatment and getting the patients on their way to the field hospital at Rouen. The battalion quartermaster was readying three wagon trains which would depart as they were filled with casualties.

"Patient survival is very much dependent on our ability to bandage their wounds, make them comfortable as possible and get them on their way. Simple as that. Now be ready."

Ashcroft motioned to James and me.

"Edwards, brief Doctor McFadden on your walk forward. You will take Corporal Ennis. McFadden, your assistant will be Corporal Timmons. Each of you will take four stretcher bearers and the line companies should have another dozen of their lads waiting to join with you."

Not a great deal of guidance I thought. I could only hope that between James and the corporal, enough information would be available to enable me to do my job.

I found Corporal Timmons near the supply tent. He was a stocky red head with a big grin. He'd already packed several ruck sacks of supplies and collected our stretcher bearers.

"My first time out there, corporal. I'm counting on you to show me what's going on and keep me from doing something stupid. Can I count on you?"

Timmons looked surprised. I couldn't tell if it was because he had just been assigned an officer who had never been at a forward aid station or because that officer had asked him to not let said officer do something stupid.

"Right, sir. I'll keep an eye on things."

"Ryan, run by the billet and grab my medical bag and my revolver. Do you have yours?"

He patted his side under his tunic.

"Good. Now off with you."

Twenty minutes later, we were looking at a map with Lieutenant Colonel Abernathy. He pointed out the present location of his companies and their respective objectives during the morning attack. He recommended two locations for aid stations, which were about one mile ahead of where our troops now held positions. James and I would be the same distance forward and 400 yards apart.

With our additional stretcher bearers, we moved out to station ourselves behind the lines of infantry, ready to advance.

The troops sat in shallow trenches, most smoking cigarettes and pipes. Each of the men had a Lee Enfield rifle close by, a harness with ammunition clips holding rounds for the rifle, a bayonet and canteen. The Highland Light Infantry crest was centered on their cap brims. All in all, they were a very impressive lot.

Checking my watch, I saw it was twenty-five minutes until the signal to advance would be sounded. The reality of what was about to happen hit me. Some of these men would possibly be under my care in the very near future, perhaps fighting for their life. I searched the faces and found myself touched by emotion. It wasn't fear or concern for them, but more a feeling of comradeship. What greater connection than men about to do battle together. I found myself wondering if my father had these feelings in South Africa. It was hard to picture my mature father as a very young doctor in a strange place and about to go into battle. But he will know what I am going through.

A loud report from our right made me jump and wheel around. More firing reports followed in what sounded like rolling thunder.

"Artillery barrage," Timmons said, with little emotion.

An average day at the hospital?

Whistles began to echo along the trench as men got up and began to move forward. Sergeants and junior officers were in front, some issuing orders, others simply moving forward.

"We follow them by one hundred yards," the corporal said and our little group moved up to the vacated trench.

The artillery fire continued unabated providing a constant level of noise blanketing the battlefield. I could only imagine what it was like where those shells were landing. That presumably was where our boys were heading.

We moved forward, our group spread out and bent down as if by signal. While there was no activity from the front, you would expect the Germans would return fire at some point. The terrain was rolling grasslands with areas of light forest. I could see farmlands to our front when we crested ridges.

Arriving at a pronounced ridge with trees dotting the slope, Corporal Timmons waved at me.

"This is a good spot, lieutenant. We can shelter the wounded on the lower part of the ridge and keep an eye on what's going on from the crest."

That made sense to me, and we began to unload our supplies.

"I'll get our bearers out after the troops know where we are."

The four teams took their orders from Timmons, picked up their stretchers and headed north toward the battalion.

"I see none of the stretcher bearers are wearing red cross armbands."

Corporal Timmons shook his head.

"No sir. It seems the German snipers like to single out bearers. No reason to help them."

"They shoot at medical teams?"

Timmons nodded.

I was glad I had my revolver. It seems this war will be much different than I imagined.

Jonesy had removed his tunic, and his revolver was in a holster on his belt. Just as well.

"Just tell me what to do," he said, sitting down next to our pile of medical supplies.

"Stick close to me, Ryan. I expect the corporal will be working by himself if we have more than one casualty at a time. I'll need assistance. Let's go through the supplies so you know what I'm asking for."

In a short time, I felt Jonesy would be able to provide enough assistance to handle the short procedures I envisioned at an aid station.

Corporal Timmons moved to the top of the ridge with a set of binoculars and was surveying to the north as the sound of gunfire ripped across the morning calm.

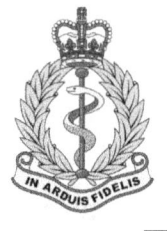

Chapter Five

"Don't worry son, I've got you."

Forward Aid Station
Near Lechelle
6 September 1914

"I see 'em." Corporal Timmons called down the slope and he left his spot on the ridge top to slide and step down to where we waited.

"One crew coming our way, didn't see anyone else. It's Jimmy Chesney's crew, good lads."

The waiting was over, it was time to take care of our wounded. But something told me I needed to get to know our stretcher bearers.

The four bearers were struggling with the stretcher as they rounded the edge of the hill. Swaying slightly, they made their way the last ten yards and lowered the soldier.

"Shot in the foot," one of the bearers said, leaning back and taking a deep breath.

"Thanks, Jimmy. What's it like up there?"

"Lot's of wounded, damned machine guns."

I saw the bloody mess of the sodier's left foot, but made my examination first.

"What's your name, son?" I asked him, his eyes wide open and face distorted with pain.

"Sullivan," he said, the pain obvious. His eyes closed and I focused on his shoe. He wore the standard high-top boot with puttees and I saw the blood oozing from around the tear in his shoe. Nothing serious as far as blood loss, he was breathing well and aware of his situation.

"Private Sullivan, once I get that shoe off and the wound bandaged, the pain will ease significantly. Ryan, cut off his puttees, while I work on the shoe."

The bullet had torn the tongue of the shoe apart, laces and all. I was able to ease the bloody shoe off his foot as Jonesy cleared the puttee.

The foot was severely damaged, but not life threatening at this point.

"I'm going to give you something for the pain, Sullivan and then these men will get you back to camp where they will take good care of you."

I bandaged the foot, the bleeding having slowed. Morphine administered, I turned him over to the bearers.

"Are you the famous Jimmy Chesney?" I asked the leader.

He looked very surprised.

"Ah, right, sir."

"I'm McFadden, glad your team is with us. I've heard good things. Can you get Private Sullivan back to camp."

"Aye, sir. Right away."

It struck me we could be easily be overwhelmed with wounded. The time it took to transport casualties by stretcher was simply too long. This is where motor-powered ambulances would make all the difference in the world.

A second bearer team arrived as the first was departing with Private Sullivan.

Again, the effort to carry a casualty a half a mile showed on the four men. Lowering the man to the ground I saw his tunic was blood soaked, the amount of blood significant. I checked for a pulse and knew he was dead. I looked up at the bearers and said, "He's gone, I'm sorry."

The reaction was not what I expected. They picked him up and moved the lad five yards away and gently set him down in the grass. Then they picked up one of the extra stretchers and headed back to the action. I wasn't sure what to make of it. They had perhaps carried a man, who was already dead, all the way back to the aid station. Were there other men they left until they returned? How do we help the bearers make a decision a man should be left until after a battle? I needed to talk with James.

"Here, he can't breathe," came the call as another crew appeared from around the hill.

These men were trotting as best they could, it was clear they felt a sense of urgency for this man.

The agonized gasp I heard as they lowered the man told me this was a true emergency. The lack of oxygen can kill a man or damage him must faster than most other problems and this man had a very short time to live if I didn't take immediate action.

"Don't worry son, I've got you," I forcefully told the wounded man.

"Does anyone know his name?"

As I conducted a quick once over, Corporal Timmons found the man's paybook in his breast pocket.

"Harry Hulswitt," Timmons said.

"All right, Harry, let's get you breathing. Ryan, open the leather case in my medical bag and lay it out here."

My surgical instruments were ready, but would I need them?

Multiple wounds covered the left side of his face and neck. My guess was a grenade or some type of shrapnel,

Leaning down I put my left hand under his neck and opened his mouth as much as possible.

"Ryan, get me a torch."

The light told me what the problem was. A piece of shrapnel had punctured the throat and was restricting the air flow. The piece of metal was the size of a shilling piece and jagged as well. The air was just making it around the right side of the throat, but I estimated it was cutting his airflow by at least three quarters.

Trying to remove the shrapnel through the throat would cause significant damage. Surgically removing it using part of the entrance wound made the most sense. It would have to do. The challenge was to avoid puncturing the jugular or carotid arteries. The initial wound had miraculously missed both. Perhaps it was God's way of telling me this man would live.

While the battalion had not included carbolic acid in the medical bag, I had my own iodine, which I felt was a better substitute than alcohol.

With Harry's throat well swabbed with iodine, I told the bearers to help Timmons hold him down.

"Ryan, you assist me."

Having performed several procedures on the trachea in London, I was comfortable that I could work my way through the neck muscles and cartilage to access the foreign body. The idea I would be doing this in an open field in France was frankly unimaginable.

"Ryan, use those gauze pads to carefully pat away the blood when I make my incision. There will be plenty of blood, don't let it bother you."

"Right."

As I made my initial incision, I knew I was doing the right thing, and could remove this. Focus was all it took.

I felt the sun on my back, odd that occurred to me, but it was summer.

Without my prompting, Jonesy patted away the initial flow of blood. Two more small incisions and I could see one side of the metal chard.

"Ryan, hand me one of those long scissor looking instruments with a pliers head on one end. The forceps."

Five minutes later the metal piece was clear of Harry's throat and we were closing the incision. While I had done this so many times, it seemed routine, Jonesy was starting transfixed as I finished up. I think my appraisal of his potential might just be right.

His tunic removed, Private Harry Hulswitt lay quietly as Jonesy dabbed his forehead with a cloth. After examining his trachea, I told Corporal Timmons that small sips of water were acceptable to get him ready for the trip back to battalion. I wanted to monitor him for at least thirty minutes to ensure there the wound had not resumed bleeding. In the meantime, we attended to the many other small fragments embedded in the side of his face.

I made sure he had morphine to keep his pain bearable and he seemed to be totally relaxed as Corporal Timmons removed the shrapnel. Why I hadn't thought about shrapnel I don't know. I assumed most wounds would be from rifle bullets. But the damage from exploding shells or grenades presented an entirely different challenge. The reality was quite sobering.

By noon, the bearers were telling us our men had taken the German defensive positions, and the enemy troops had retreated to the north. Our total for the day so far was seventeen soldiers at the aid station. Fourteen had been sent back to battalion while the bodies of three lay to one side, covered by blankets. Now what, I wondered? Does someone order us to fall back or move forward. Was there some procedure or protocol for the culmination of an attack.

I sat down and drank some water. My back hurt from leaning over patients, but I realized I felt overwhelmed by what I had seen that morning. In London, my encounters with the human body were most clinical and in a very controlled environment. This morning, all I had seen was men whose bodies had been assaulted, whether by bullet or shell. They had lain in dirt under a hot sun, their blood soaking through their uniforms. I was very tired. This is not what I expected.

A runner from Major Ashcroft found us at 4:00pm. Our orders were to return to the battalion aid station in preparation for the entire battalion moving forward first thing in the morning.

As we packed our medical sacks, I asked Corporal Timmons what should we do with the three soldiers who lay in the grass next to us?

"That's why we brought the shovels, sir. The lads and I will dig graves for them. I'll copy their names in me book and give 'em to the adjutant. You and Private Jones head back to camp and we'll follow."

Corporal Timmons face was covered with dirt, sweat and a smear of blood. He was probably in his late twenties, but looked much older. It had been a long day for him and certainly for the stretcher bearers.

"Let's all get busy, corporal," I said, picking up a shovel and walking over to the three soldiers lying under the blankets. I saw that Jimmy Chesney had picked up a shovel and walked behind us with his team.

Lifting each blanket, I looked at each soldier's identity disc. Privates Ian Brown, Jerimiah Colton and Leslie Carnes were about to be buried in the soil of France. I wondered if they would ever be recovered to be sent back to England. Then it struck me how impossible that would be. The men that went to war, in many cases, were off to ultimate oblivion. But I suppose that was the way of war.

All of us turned to digging three graves. There was little said while we dug, all of us with our own thoughts. This was the way of war I was starting to understand. When it came time, we covered the lads with what we had in the way of sheeting. Then filled in the graves.

When we finished, I wished I had something religious to say, but knew I didn't.

"Go with God," I said, and the other men answered with "Amen."

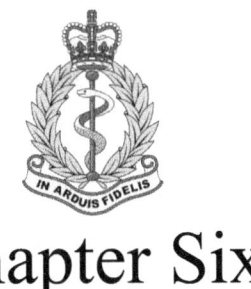

Chapter Six

"Our machine guns are very smooth."

2nd Battalion Bivouac
North of Meaux
6 September 1914

Arriving back at camp, I felt truly exhausted. During the thirty-minute hike back to camp, the men were quiet. Everyone seemed to be putting one foot in front of the other, with little banter or anticipation of food and rest. But my thoughts returned to those wounded men. It was like they were coming in from a queue. One after the other, torn, bleeding and in shock. This was war?

The medical area was in the process of being broken down, tents coming down and trunks being packed.

"Corporal Timmons, thank you," I said and extended my hand.

He seemed surprised and took my hand tentatively.

"It went all right, sir."

"Can you replenish our supplies in case we go out tomorrow?"

"Well, yes, sir."

"I want you with me, Corporal Timmons. If you see that not happening, you come find me."

He grinned.

"Aye, sir. I'll do that."

"And corporal, what is your first name?"

"Corey, sir."

"Corey, a good Scottish name. Good night"

At my shelter, I found James, sitting on a wooden crate, taking off his left shoe.

"Getting ready for a nice soak, I'll wager."

He looked up.

"David, you survived your first day."

I sat down on the ground in front of him.

"Good lord, I'm a complete novice. No idea what was going on, but Corporal Timmons took care of me."

"He's a good man. Should be a sergeant if you ask me."

James began massaging his ankle.

"What's with your ankle?"

"Twisted the damn thing on my way back here. Not sprained but damned sore."

"Let the doctor provide some relief."

Going through my gear, I pulled out my bottle of scotch and a metal cup.

"Got a cup?"

James pulled a ceramic mug from his rucksack.

Drinks poured, I raised my glass.

"To those we lost today."

He raised his glass.

"To the lads."

"James, we've all seen death. But today was different. Those lads were healthy young men. Not some sick disease ridden geriatric in a London hospital."

James smiled.

"I've been told it's a difficult thing to keep your humanity as the casualties mount. Let's face it, all of them are young with their lives in front of them. But we can't let it overwhelm us. How we accomplish that, I'm not sure, but we have to try."

Jonesy walked up, carrying my bag over his shoulder.

"Everything replaced including your iodine. Corporal Timmons helped me."

"Thank you, Ryan. By the way, would you see if you can locate a field notebook like Corporal Timmons was carrying. I think we'll need one.

"Aye, doc."

A soldier approached our shelter with a torch lighting his way.

"I'm looking for Doctor McFadden."

"I'm McFadden."

"Sir, the battalion commander would like to see you and he asks that you to bring your medical bag."

I found Lieutenant Colonel Abernathy in a small field tent, lying on a canvas cot. His tunic was off, and his shirt was blood-stained on his right side.

"McFadden here sir, you asked for me?"

"Come in," he said. A pillow and blanket supported his head, allowing him to look at me as we spoke.

"As you can see, I have a small problem. I decided someone should take a look at it."

"Of course, sir."

I put my bag down and moved to his side.

"When did this happen?"

"Midday as I recall. Stung mightily, but I knew it wasn't serious."

"May I?" I asked, reaching down to unbutton his shirt.

"Please, yes."

As I gently pulled on the shirt, it was clear the blood had dried and the shirt now adhered to the wound,

"I'll have my assistant get some warm water to dissolve the blood."

Stepping out of the tent I told Jonesy what I needed.

Back with the colonel, I saw his eyes were closed. He grimaced then opened his eyes.

"Your father was Lennox McFadden?"

Hearing my father's name surprised me and I nodded.

"Yes, sir, of Glasgow."

"And formerly of the Highland Light Infantry?"

Now I was curious. How could he know this?

"Yes, sir, he was."

Abernathy smiled.

"He was our regimental surgeon during the Boer campaign. He removed a Boer rifle bullet from my leg in January of 1900. I got to know you father well during my recovery."

The warm water took care of the caked-on blood and I was able to pull the shirt free of the wound. A large flap of skin and tissue had been torn from the colonel's side as a bullet grazed his body. An inch or two over and this would be an entirely different problem or even a fatality.

"I'll clean the wound, then suture it closed. I would recommend an abdominal bandage to reduce the tension on the stitches for at least two days."

"We'll resume our attack in the morning, but I will try to keep my activity to a minimum."

"I can check on you in the morning and after the attack tomorrow."

"Only if you don't have other pressing duties. Where were you today?"

I gathered up my instruments and handed the bag to Jonesy.

"In a forward aid station, sir."

"How did it go?"

"My first time, sir. But it seemed to proceed well. Corporal Timmons certainly kept me in line."

Abernathy laughed.

"Our non-commissioned officers are the backbone of the battalion. We're lucky to have such an experienced group. Some of the senior sergeants were with me in Africa."

The colonel carefully swung his feet over and down to the floor of the tent.

"Thank you, doctor. It seems one more time, an Abernathy has been taken care of by a McFadden. A bit of tradition, I think."

I smiled.

"Yes, sir."

There was a call from outside the tent.

"Colonel?"

Abernathy replied, "Come in, please."

A slim office in his mid-30's entered.

"Doctor, this is my second in command, Major Bennett.

We shook hands.

"Colonel, here are the reports you wanted."

It appeared my presence was no longer required, and I excused myself. Good Lord, is this what the war was like. Men die and we have a drink and then clean up things and go to bed?

The morning was a repeat of the previous day. The line companies were mustering as James, and I made our way to meet Major Ashcroft.

My check of the battalion commander had taken only a moment as he hurried away with several of his staff members including Major Bennett. Colonel Abernathy assured me his rest was sufficient, and the pain was quite manageable.

"Abernathy's a good man," James said as we worked our way across camp. I hear he can be found much closer to the action than most other senior officers."

"That's likely why he was wounded yesterday," I commented.

"By the way, unless you want to see him lose his rag, don't mention to Ashcroft that you treated the battalion commander."

No doubt the major would have considered treating Abernathy as his right or due in the military way of things. It seemed quite normal to me, particularly with the unique connection. But my friend was right, no sense in poking the bear."

"What's the story on Major Bennett?"

James said, "Good man, regular army.   He was a company commander before the war, keeps all of the paperwork and supplies flowing. We're lucky to have a top rate one and two."

A good situation I thought.

"Ah, there you are."

We both saluted the major and waited for his words of wisdom.

"Same plan today, gentlemen. The forward aid stations should be in the area close to the German positions yesterday. Hopefully there will be some type of shelter you'll be able to use."

We nodded.

"Edwards, you make sure the personnel are ready to move out. Doctor McFadden, walk with me."

I followed him toward a small copse of trees. Reaching the trees, he turned and assumed a position much like 'at ease" with both feet at shoulder width, hand in the small of his back.

"It was very evident as I examined the wounded coming in from you air station that you performed at least two procedures that should have been left to medical teams in the rear."

For a moment, I thought I had heard him incorrectly. In both cases, the procedures took less than twenty minutes. I was able to ease the pain for Private Sullivan and hell, Harry Hulswit would have died if I hadn't intervened. What was this fool talking about?

"You are to expedite the movement of wounded back to the battalion aid station where the medical staff can deal with them in a thorough and professional manner, clear?"

Remembering what James had said about Ashcroft being a problem, I fought my urge to tell him what I really thought.

"Ah, yes, sir. I understand."

I looked at him but said nothing else.

Ashcroft looked like he was expecting more of a response from me, but then my silence seemed to confuse him.

"Right, quite right," he said and turned on his heel, walking back to the medical area.

Standing there I decided to continue to provide the best care I could, keeping in mind what the major had said, but I was not going to pass wounded along, if my care would provide a better outcome.

The move to our new aid station, located in a partially destroyed house, took almost an hour. I wondered how far we had to advance before the battalion bivouac would move forward. This distance was going to be a challenge to our bearers, to say nothing of severely wounded men. If the journey back took thirty minutes, the men available to carry new wounded could be all on their way back to battalion.

Corporal Timmons told me that the line companies did have stretchers and could draft men as bearers if needed. But in the confusion of battle, it simply made the task of moving men to the rear much more difficult.

For the first time our location was close enough to hear very vividly the gunfire of the assault and return fire of the Germans. In the midst of rifle volley fire, the staccato of machine gun fire was more and more evident.

"Vickers," Corporal Timmons said after one long burst. "Our machine guns are very smooth."

Just then we heard another burst that sounded different.

I looked at the corporal.

"German Maxim 08," he said, "More rhythmic."

My God, I thought, what else will I learn before this is

over?

As the bearers headed out I called after them.

"Keep you heads down, boys,"

Jimmy Chesney looked back grinning.

"Will do, doc."

Twenty minutes later, Jimmy's team arrived with a soldier, his lower face swathed in bloody bandages. Several individual medical kits must have been emptied to come up with that much gauze.

I cut off the bandages and saw that the man's jaw had been shattered on the right side. The structural support was gone and the soft tissue was severely damaged. He was breathing, but with labor and I carefully examined his mouth. Tissue and teeth were hampering the air flow, and I opened the airway by removing both.

"Morphine," I told Jonesy, not seeing any evidence that he had been administered the pain killer.

"Don't try to talk, son. Let me clean this up and we'll have you on your way to hospital right away.

"Ryan, cut away his webbing and open his tunic."

We could cool him down and make him more comfortable for the litter carry back to battalion. The best I could do was reapply a more effective bandage. He was going to have a very tough go of it. Half his lower jaw was essentially gone. I had seen some reconstructive surgery in London, but at best, the functionality of the mouth might be restored. The poor lad would be horribly disfigured for the rest of his life.

"Do you need water," I asked him, knowing the heat, dust and blood must be horrible.

His eyes said it all, but he nodded.

I pulled out my handkerchief.

"Ryan, get me a cup of water, and his name."

Soaking the cloth, I carefully moved the boy's head and then dripped water on his tongue. No choking and he nodded his head again. Several more squeezes and I laid his head back down. I patted his leg.

"You're going to be fine, Lowell."

As the afternoon wore on, the flow of wounded was steady. Our sense of the battle was an ebb and flow, with small advances followed by pulling back to defended positions. The German machine guns were proving to be particular problems as it appeared the units opposing our men had a greater number of the Maxims compared to our Vickers. According to Corporal Timmons, our machine gun company was equipped with only two of the Vickers.

The reality of the damage from the machine guns came home to us when a soldier arrived with his left leg, arm and shoulder all having been hit by a German machine gun. The wounds appeared to resemble the normal rifle bullet wounds, but multiple wounds compounded the threat to the young man.

Jonesy helped get his webbing and tunic off while the man reacted slightly. It was clear he was going into shock.

"Ryan, get his feet elevated while I tighten the bandages on his wounds."

If we could reduce his blood loss, he might have a chance.

Whoever initially bandaged him actually did a good job and I simply reinforced the bandages on his arm and shoulder. I applied a tourniquet high on his leg as it was the most significant bleeder.

The pale face told me it was not going well for him. His pulse was also rapid and weak.

"Let's move him into the shade and I want you to take a wet rag and wipe down his face, neck and hands."

I wanted to see if we could let his body catch up and stabilize before trying to send him back to battalion.

An officer came around the remaining wall of the house and I immediately saw he was a chaplain. A big man, he moved rather gracefully.

"Hello, Hello," he said walking up and kneeling down to extend his hand.

"Father Michael Gallagher, doctor," he said grinning, "Out to see the lads."

"Welcome, father." I was Church of Scotland, but knew many Catholics in Glasgow. Anything that might help these men deal with their injuries was welcome by me.

"Corporal John Livesay," Jonesy said, the break in treatment giving him time to find the man's paybook.

Chaplain Gallagher went down on the other knee and make the sign of the cross, closed his eyes and appeared to by saying a prayer.

"Amen," he said opening his eyes.

As the sound of battle rose to a crescendo, two more litters arrived in quick succession. I quickly checked both men and satisfied myself that while painful, neither wound was immediately life threatening. Both men suffered bullet wounds, one in the hand another in the thigh. Cleaning, bandaging and morphine were taken care of and the men given water.

"What can I do to help?" Father Gallagher asked.

He honestly looked like he wanted to help, so I handed him a canvas bucket.

"Father, we're low on water. There's a well about fifty yards down that street."

Grinning at me he took the bucket and said, "Righto."

That was my introduction to Michael Francis Gallagher, whom I later learned to call "padre." Over the afternoon I watched while he assisted our little group with every task. He demonstrated that he was a humble man, who was here to serve his God and the regiment. Despite the difficulty of seeing the wounded men, he ignored the blood, pain and terror to provide a calming spirit. As he assisted, he would speak with the wounded men as if they were in church. I found it surprisingly soothing myself as I went about my business.

By late afternoon, we had seen twenty men, of which two died before they could move on to battalion. I watched the padre administer the last rites to a catholic soldier and a just as compassionate prayer for the other lad. It reinforced my faith in the goodness of man, despite the current horror we were witnessing. My learning was continuing at a rather rapid pace.

My second day was not any easier. While I was able to provide the clinical care for the wounded men, I found myself mentally exhausted. The never-ending parade of bleeding and suffering men was something I could not ignore. How do physicians, orderlies, nurses, whomever cares for these men keep their sanity? I shall do my very best to do my duty, that is what will keep me taking care of them. That is all I can do.

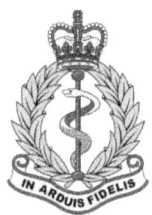

Chapter Seven

"I have prepared a letter of reprimand."

2nd Battalion Bivouac
South of the Aisne River
2 October 1914

When you read of the battles and campaigns of the past, it is hard to get a sense of the all-encompassing experience a protracted battle provides. Over the last two weeks, the French and ourselves had steadily advanced north pushing the Germans back toward Belgium. At the same time, a push by our left flank attempted to drive to the sea and turn the German flank. The results were not spectacular, but we were able to hold the enemy in place. Paris was now safe and while we did not recapture Antwerp, the French channel ports were out of the line of fire.

At the time, I felt the advance was terribly bloody, the number of casualties building every day. Perhaps we were fortunate that as the intensity of fighting increased, we were able to adjust our work to handle the increased number of wounded and the continuing complication of bursting artillery shells. The use of machine guns increased in short order. Our machine gun company receiving more of the Vickers Mark 1 guns. The scale of what was happening struck us as the total number of killed and wounded in the three years of the Boer War was 30,000 men. During our advance on the Aisne River, we have suffered 13,000 killed wounded and missing. Missing, there is a strange category. I could never understand how anyone could be missing. But now I understand as human bodies disappear when high explosive shells detonate. Soldiers are buried on site or there are only pieces of flesh that end up being buried. The chaos will only continue to produce more and more missing. What do we tell their families?

Our original protective dugouts began a transformation to a series of reinforced trenches as the lines stabilized. At the time we thought this was going to be an intermediate step as we re-grouped for the next big push. What we didn't understand was that the German's supply lines had now caught up with their front lines. On the other side, the enemy also was constructing more permanent defensive positions. Without our realizing it, the war had changed.

In a very short period of time, we had become veterans as it were. The daily attacks, re-supply, artillery barrages and the business of staying alive became second nature. I was continually impressed at how our stretcher bearers rose to the challenge.

Of particular note, I watched Ryan Jones continue to undergo a remarkable transition from dispatch rider to valuable medical assistant. His interest in all things medical was encouraging to me while at the same time intrusive as he would invariably ask a question at a key moment in a procedure. But he never seemed discouraged even when I was sharp with him. He also took his turn with the stretcher bearers when the work load was light. The lingering question for me was how long before someone came looking for him?

In an area near the main battalion medical area, Jonesy and Corey Timmons took charge of making a semi-protected dugout for myself and James Edwards. While not truly underground, the area we slept in was in a dug out area, with wooden boards for a floor. A canvas covering provided protection from the rain.

An area fifty yards behind the main defensive trench was built up as an aid station where a doctor was stationed during the day and a medical orderly at other times. If a patrol was going out, the aid station was fully manned. A large patrol would mean an aid team including a doctor would move forward to the main trench to be immediately available to the returning patrol.

For the second day, we had no casualties in the aid station. Both sides were recovering from the last two weeks' battle and there was a lull in rifle and machine gun fire along the trench lines. with a lack of artillery shell impacts led to a first time visit to our little piece of the front.

Major Ashcroft arrived, with no notice, accompanied by Sergeant Loeffler.

Corporal Timmons and I were brewing up a cookpot of water for tea. Four of our bearers sat smoking and talking among themselves, while four more were fast asleep at the back of the dugout. Jonesy had his head down cleaning my surgical instruments after he boiled them in the sterile pot.

"Hello McFadden, I thought it was time to conduct an inspection. We certainly don't want to see our standards go down."

I stood up and saluted Ashcroft, who returned my salute and looked around our area.

"Looks like everyone is on make and mend, eh?"

"Sir, I gave the bearers permission to sleep. There's no need for them at the moment and they've been up at all hours these last two weeks." I knew Ashcroft never missed a meal or a good night's sleep back at the bivouac.

"Right," he said, his disapproval clear in his tone.

"We're making some tea sir, would you care for some?"

"Uh, no thank you. What's that man doing?" He asked, pointing to Jonesy.

"He's cleaning surgical instruments, sir."

"Even though you have been told that surgery in the field is discouraged?"

Corporal Timmons and Jonesy both looked up.

"Major, might we talk outside?"

"Of course."

I was ready to let Ashcroft know what I thought of his intent, when he pre-empted me.

"Lieutenant, you know my policy about elective surgery in the field. You have continually violated that policy over the last two weeks. It was clear to me as I saw your telltale iodine covering men and saw the attached notes."

My anger began to take over and I began to make my point when he interrupted me.

"Your oath of allegiance states that you will obey all orders of officers set over you. You have most certainly not done that. For that reason, I have prepared a letter of reprimand for the colonel's signature. For now, I will recommend you remain on duty in the field, but the next time you will find yourself marching to the rear to count pills in some warehouse. Is that clear?"

As much as I wanted to tell him what I thought, common sense prevailed.

"Yes, sir."

That afternoon I made up my mind to take things into my own hands. If the army wanted me to practice institutional medicine, they could damn well throw me out. The hell with them.

I found the battalion commander's tent and asked if he was available. Everyone knew me from my visits to check on the colonel's wound two weeks ago.

"Hello, doctor."

"Good afternoon, colonel. Might I talk with you?"

"Is this official business as opposed to medical?"

He had me on that one.

"A bit of both, sir."

"Let me get ahead of you on this. I just read a letter from Major Ashcroft reprimanding you for violating his verbal orders. Is that true?"

The charge sounded cut and dry, but then it was.

"Yes, sir, I did."

His relaxed demeanor changed slightly, and I felt the previous doctor patient relationship had vanished.

"Do you know why it is so important to follow orders?"

I didn't have a set answer, so I took a stab.

"Because it is the only way an army can work."

"That is true, for the most part. But a key part of that is that you may not have all of the information that a superior has which supports what he is ordering."

I looked back, feeling a bit less sure of myself.

"I can see that, sir."

"And ultimately men's lives depend upon it."

"That's my point, sir. His orders put some men at risk of death or more serious effects from their wounds."

Colonel Abernathy sat back and looked hard at me.

"Explain yourself, lieutenant."

Later that evening I was back in the colonel's tent, accompanied by Major Ashcroft. I immediately noticed the colonel was wearing his tunic, sitting at the small platform he used for a desk. We both stood.

"Lieutenant, it appears to me that you have had some trouble adjusting to the way the army does things. I'm here to remind you that it is your duty to follow the orders of those senior to you. Do you understand me?"

I didn't understand. When I left earlier, he seemed to realize that what I was doing was helping to save the lives of his men. Now he was berating me, in front of the senior medical officer.

"Yes, sir. I…"

"There is nothing else to say, lieutenant. You are dismissed."

With an about turn, I left the tent, having had my thrashing.

"Well, he could have court-martialed you," James said. "Look at the positive side. You won't have to give up these palatial surroundings, gourmet meals and life of relaxation."

I did smile, but still felt like my father had just given me a hiding.

"I'm going to take a walk."

Major Bennett came around the latrine, making a direct line for our dugout.

"Doctor, do you have a moment?"

I saluted.

"Yes, sir, certainly."

Another tongue lashing?

"I just wanted to say that I think you have been doing a fine job."

"Ah, yes, sir, thank you."

"You know I handle most of the administrative work for the battalion?"

"Yes, sir, I did."

"Well, here is a letter I think should be destroyed. But I will leave that up to you."

Confused, I said, "Yes, sir."

"Have a good night," the major said, walking into the darkness.

I stepped back into the dugout and opened the letter. It was the letter from Major Ashcroft to the colonel about my activities. Smiling, I tucked the letter in my tunic and left to continue my walk.

Seeing Jonesy at the end of the dugout line, I walked down and sat down on the sandbag next to him.

"Ready for tomorrow?" I asked.

"All set."

"How are you doing?"

He turned towards me.

"Me?"

"This has been a hard two weeks. Are you getting on all right?"

"Truth be, I feel like I'm doing sumin' important."

"Feels good, doesn't it?" I said.

"Aye, does. Jus' worryn' bout what my company's thinking, maybe I'm dead or deserted."

Good Lord, I never thought of that.

"Have you written your family?"

He shook his head,

"Don't have family. Raised by 'n uncle, but he died last year."

His company might be carrying him missing or deserted. I must get this sorted. Or else.

"Ryan, let me take care of this. The fact is that you've been a great help, and I don't want to lose you."

"You're telling the truth?"

"Indeed I am. You've taken to medicine quite well."

He smiled and said, "Could you teach me more?"

"I would be happy to do so."

The instruction of Ryan Jones would be my winter project.

"Doctor McFadden."

I looked up to see Major Ashcroft walking toward me as I was packing a medical haversack.

Coming to attention, I saluted.

"Sir."

"I have been giving a great deal of thought to our disagreements over the use of surgery in the field."

His tone was casual, and I wondered where this could possibly be going.

"Yes, sir."

"Certainly, I understand how some procedures are beneficial in certain circumstances. Perhaps we should make some provision for straightforward surgical procedures when time and situation allow."

Damn, it sounds like the colonel must have had words with him after I left.

"Yes, sir. I see your point."

"Moving forward, I expect you to exercise good judgement, but if you feel a procedure is called for, proceed if the situation will allow you."

This was remarkable, I thought. Use your head McFadden, this is an opportunity.

"Sir, perhaps until I have a better feel for your guidance, I could give you a debrief of my field procedures to see if you concur with my actions."

Ashcroft nodded.

"That is a splendid idea, doctor. We shall do just that."

I decided not to tell him that I burned his letter last night.

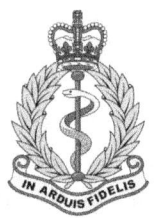

Chapter Eight

"...the cold weather seemed to intensify the ongoing battle with lice."

2nd Battalion Bivouac
South of the Aisne River
20 November 1914

The first several weeks into November became a probing and feeling out time for both sides. Patrols would venture out at night, feeling their way toward the enemy lines, taking note of defenses. In short order, we also saw wire parties, from both sides installing barbed wire to protect the trench positions. By November, the areas between the German and Allied lines were being referred to an "No Man's Land."

The conditions began to be truly awful. Cold weather brought on an increase in colds, fevers, coughs and a curse of all armys, trench foot. Freezing rain and sleet kept the troops constantly wet and mud became a challenge I could have never imagined. Not only were the men covered in the glutinous mess, but some were actually became stuck. Cave ins were common and soon having wooden duckboards on the trench bottoms became a matter of safety, not just comfort.

The infantry began using barbed wire to channel any attacking troops into fire zones where machine guns were set up to deliver a withering fire The trench systems slowly became more and more complex. Communication trenches would connect fighting trenches and living dugouts. At night the unsuspecting soldier could easily find himself lost in a bewildering maze of dirt and mud.

By this time, we had also become used to seeing aircraft overhead and many were German. The Royal Flying Corps was also present and providing reconnaissance. The use of aircraft and telephones on the battlefield raised the level of continual intensity that had never been seen in warfare before. While battles in the past might have been weeks or months apart, now the infantrymen were in contact with the enemy at all times. The effect on men over time was something no one had anticipated. As the use of artillery barrages became more common, the constance pressure on the men in the trenches took a terrible toll. But again, it took time for us to recognize it, much to our shame.

As we moved from November to December, our staff confirmed the Germans were entrenching their artillery behind, in some cases, three lines of trenches. The battleground had become static in a very short time and the armies seemed to pause their efforts while the commanders decided how to proceed.

It was during the fall that we learned to appreciate the ability of the German artillery. As we occupied more permanent locations, the artillery began to search out our key positions. We learned the value of sandbags, timber and camouflage. From a positive standpoint, having known locations of company areas, supply sites, aid stations and even latrines made daily operations much more efficient.

The other realization was the rapid onset of winter. Fall had been brief, and lower temperatures were upon us. High temperatures barely made it into the 50's while nighttime temperatures slid into the low 40's. The wool favored by the army for uniforms became much more pleasant, particularly the greatcoats that covered men below their knees.

The other problem which rapidly dawned upon us was the rains and natural water capture by our trenches. Soon the men were dealing with mud, which coated everything and within a month we saw our first cases of immersion foot. We were able to get a good supply of army issue foot powder, but getting the men to use it was another thing. The demand for extra socks also took the quartermasters by surprise. It was clear we needed to spearhead foot hygiene or our foot soldiers weren't going to be able to use their feet.

By December, a system of troop rotation was established. Five or six days in the forward trenches were followed by a week or so in the reserve trenches located several hundred yards behind the front. After a week in the reserve trenches, the platoon would move to a bivouac area where they could bath, get clean clothes, seek routine medical attention and try to regain their strength. In short order, the army provided the support we needed in the way of tentage, spare uniforms, portable stoves and construction material. The onset of the cold weather provided an extra impetus for construction of shelters that could provide reasonable protection for our men.

Unfortunately, the cold weather seemed to intensify the ongoing battle with lice. Any time in the trenches would guarantee lice infestation in short order. While on site attempts to deal with the parasite invariably failed, a rotation back to the rest area complete with a thorough disinfecting would at least give the men temporary relief. My personal efforts failed, and I took my turn in the disinfecting process.

By Christmas, a routine of sorts developed. Occasional patrols were the only active military activity by the battalion. Some of the officers took leave, returning to England for a week or ten days providing a break from the dreariness of the front. Other ranks were also allowed to take leave if the operational tempo allowed it. The ongoing stress and demands of living in the elements affected every man differently. Some withdrew into themselves, others made no bones about the harsh conditions, while others seemed to take it all in stride. I must say that my overcoat and a dry dugout kept me in reasonable spirits, despite the lice. The challenge of getting to England and back was not something I wanted to deal with and so I chose not to request a leave. Perhaps in the new year.

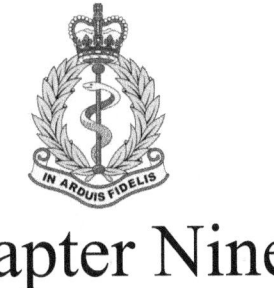

Chapter Nine

"I put a circular bandage around his head to hold everything in place."

2nd Battalion Bivouac
Southwest of Neuve Chapelle
9 March 1915

Tension was palpable across the camp, with plans for the attack tomorrow now known. The dreary months of January and February had given way to a tactical resetting of the BEF and preparation for the first offensive move of the war. As I understood it, the high command felt a surprise assault, coupled with a significant artillery barrage would allow our troops to break through the German defenses. Once breached, more troops would pour through and expand into the enemy's rear area.

We had seen some of the new heavy guns making their way to their emplacements. The 18 pounders were expected to destroy the German's defensive wire positions allowing our troop to attack the enemy's trenches directly. Told our objective was the town of Neuve Chapelle I realized I didn't care. I knew whatever place we were trying to capture, our men would die and suffer wounds. I guess I would never make a great general.

The ferocity of the barrage was something I could have never imagined. Multiple batteries of guns fired shell after shell at the German lines. We were told some of the shells would be aimed at the wire barriers to cut a path through for our men. Sitting in our makeshift aid station one mile from the artillery's impact area, you could feel the concussion of the shells. What must it be like for the Germans or even our men just two to three hundred yards away?

As the barrage came to an end, we knew our troops would be attacking. Our bearers understood and moved out toward the front. We checked our equipment and waited.

Thirty minutes later the first bearer team arrived, carrying a man with a gunshot wound in the shoulder. That was straightforward, but what the team described was not. The barrage had not destroyed the wire nor the German trenches. Our first attack was decimated. Now there were many wounded in No Man's Land but the battle continued.

"Corporal, finish bandaging this man's shoulder. I'm going to go up and see what I can do."

This was not what aid station medical officers were expected to do, but the truth be known, sending our bearer teams out time after time had made me feel I was shirking the real danger. I needed to know what it was like.

"Ryan, do you have your pistol."

He nodded.

"Grab two medical packs," I said.

"Yes, sir." He sounded quite formal and stilted for some reason.

"What can I do?" came a question from behind me. It was Chaplain Gallagher.

The idea struck me. The Chaplain had been sitting in on many of my sessions with Jonesy and now possessed a fair working knowledge of advanced first aid and battlefield dressings.

"Padre, I need you to stay here with the corporal and handle whatever might come in. I'm going out to see if we can get any of the wounded back to our trenches."

Gallagher said, "I'll be happy to help the corporal."

"Thank you, chaplain. Ryan, let's go."

Moving toward the battle, I could see smoke and hear the ongoing thunder of rifle and machine gun fire. Our trench line was the first obstacle, and we found one of our teams taking cover beneath the overhang of a wooden parapet.

"Jimmy's out there," the team leader, a private named Golden, said.

The firing seemed to intensify, then drop off.

"I'll move forward and see if I can contact Jimmy or find any wounded. Follow me in two minutes and stay as low as you can."

Was this foolish? Just, go.

I reached out and began climbing the ladder. As my eyes reached the top of the trench, I saw a devastated landscape. Large shell holes spread across No Man's Land. Wire barriers were immediately to my front. Dust and smoke drifted across the torn earth. For a moment I froze, not sure what to do. Then I reached out, grabbed dirt and began crawling toward the first large crater. The recent rains left the ground slippery and beneath the surface, mud oozed up. A rifle shot cracked overhead, the sound terrifying as I knew there was no place to shelter. I had to make it to the shell crater. Almost like a swimmer, I moved my arms and legs, trying to stay as close to the earth as humanly possible. In another minute I reached the edge of the crater and pulled myself over into the pit.

Sliding nose down, I hit a pool of water at the bottom of the crater.

My God, this is insane I thought. A burst of machine gun fire cracked over my crater, but I had no idea if it was ours or the German's. Getting up on my elbows I looked into the eyes of a dead British private. The entire side of his chest including his arm was missing. His face showed a surprised look, but his eyes were vacant.

I got on my haunches as Jonesy came over the edge. He slid down the side, hitting me and driving us both into the water.

"Christ!" I expelled and blew foul putrid water out of my mouth,

"Sorry," Jonesy said as we both scrambled back on the dry side of the crater.

Another burst of automatic fire made us lay back, our hands holding us out of the water.

"Mother Mary," Jonesy said.

"Hold on, Jonesy, hold on."

We lay there, neither saying a word.

At that moment, Private Golden came over the edge of the crater, dragging a stretcher, followed in close order by the rest of his team.

"Sir!" Golden said as the team gathered themselves.

Trying to use logic at this point was probably futile, but it was the only thing I could think of.

"All right. Jonesy and I will move forward and go into the next big craters. If we find any of our lads, we'll call to you. Come up and we'll try to get them out."

The second crawl didn't seem so bad. I moved left around a tangle of barbed wire, torn up by artillery. Ahead of me another large crater beckoned. Pulling myself over the side, I slide down and stopped, looking across at two of our boys. Pulling myself across the water in the bottom, I reached the two who were side by side, face down.

Quickly checking, both had faint and rapid pulses. There was a great deal of blood on both of their tunics. I rolled the first man over and saw two entry wounds, one on his upper torso left and then one right. Good for now.

Rolling the second man over, he had a wound directly below his ribcage which likely had torn his abdomen apart. I reached down and unbuttoned his tunic as he regained some degree of consciousness.

"What…" he cried, reaching into the air.

"Relax, son, I've got you."

The blood soaked his trousers and when I cut them open, I saw his intestines protruding from a horizontal tear. More firing crashed overhead as I looked at the shiny bowels, steam rising from the wound. Dear God, I thought this boy can't survive this wound. Not lying in a shell crater in the middle of nowhere. In London, in an operating room, I could try to save him, but not here.

I found his paybook. "John Shilling, Private."

He gasped, the pain now taking control.

"Stay with me, John," I said. I opened my medical satchel. Reaching for the morphine injectables, I injected one in his thigh, then another, knowing he would slip away.

"Rest easy, son."

What had I just done? Was I now part of the machine allowing this insanity to continue? No, there was no choice. If it was me, I would want the same. Perhaps I had lost my humanity as this carnage continued. But I didn't have the luxury of reflection.

I turned to his mate and opened the tunic after cutting his web gear.

The wounds were not simple, but also not life-threatening.

"What's your name?"

"Paul Howard."

"Just lay back, Paul. I'm going to bandage your chest, then Private Golden and his team will get you to the rear."

Jonesy was already preparing bandages and cutting Howard's shirt for better access.

Ten minutes had Paul Howard ready for transport.

"Private Golden, get Howard to the rear when able. Jonesy and I are going to move up and see if we can locate Jimmy and his crew."

"Right, doc. Are you sure you want to do that?"

With more bravado than I felt, I said, "Can't fix them if we can't find them. You be careful on your way back."

He nodded then we both ducked as a shell detonated near us. Dirt, rock and shreds of wire landed around us, but no one was hurt.

I checked John Shilling. He was gone. Looking at that young face, I wanted to scream that this was insane. But whomever might hear me knew that. The world had changed.

"Ryan, let's move."

We located Jimmy Chesney and his bearers about one hundred feet ahead. The crater they had taken refuge in was deeper than most others and four wounded men were sharing the shell hole.

"We brought 'em all here when the shelling started up," Jimmy yelled, another shell exploding in the distance.

Four wounded, one stretcher.

Quickly as I could, I examined each man. Jonesy was at my side, getting names and helping me get past their tunics, webbing and trousers.

Two looked like they would be able to walk themselves back to our trenches. We quickly bandaged their wounds, which painful, were not serious.

A third soldier had been shot through the left side of his abdomen. He was in extreme pain and I administered morphine, knowing he would need the stretcher.

The last soldier had been shot in the head. What looked like a glancing impact had torn a piece of skull off down to the dura. Amazingly, the dura looked intact through the blood and hair. Carefully covering the wound with gauze pads, I put a circular bandage around his head to hold everything in place.

In the back of my mind I realized there had not been any shells exploding in the last ten minutes. Was this a chance to get back to our lines?

"Jimmy, can you strap our abdominal wound down?"

"Aye, we can."

"Get ready to move." I told the group. "Ryan, you'll take charge of our two walking wounded. And bring one of their rifles, we might need it."

I had decided I could carry our headwound. He looked lighter than most soldiers and I had always been able to carry weight.

"Leave anything we don't need," I told them, and let's go."

Climbing out of the crater was the first challenge and Jonesy led the effort. He lifted and helped his two wards over the lip and was gone.

"Jimmy, follow me," I said, kneeling down and putting the young soldier over my right shoulder. One of Jimmy's bearers helped me up the side of the crater and over the side. Once on flat terrain, I was able to balance the weight and follow Jonesy and his patients.

Random rifle shots rang out as we moved rearward. I don't think they were aimed at us, but I tried to move faster. During the fifteen minutes it took us to cross No Man's Land, there was no artillery activity. I think God was giving us a pass.

It had been many years since I had spent time on serious exercise and by the time I reached our first trench, I was done. Sliding into the trench, I let soldiers take over my burden and slid to the floor. My uniform was torn, filthy and bloody. But I felt like I was part of the men in a different way from the aid station. I knew what it was like and I was able to bring our casualties to safety. The two walking wounded sat on a dirt ledge, drinking water. I saw Jimmy lead his team to the edge of trench and watched the men wrestle the stretcher down.

Rolling on my knees, I had to check on the abdominal wound.

"What's this?"

I looked up to see the battalion commander and his assistant. Lieutenant Colonel Abernathy's uniform was streaked with mud and his face grimy.

"Bringing in some casualties, sir."

I got to my feet.

"If you'll excuse me, sir."

I knelt over the stretcher.

"Does anyone have a medical pouch? We had to leave ours out there."

My patient needed morphine and for once I had been caught without my supply. Thank goodness he appeared to be solidly conscious, although clearly in pain.

"Here, doc."

There were no injectables, but thank the Lord there were morphine pills.

After administering the pills, I moved over to the head wound. Abernathy was next to the young soldier, who was still unconscious.

"I think we were lucky her, sir. While he lost some skull, the dura was intact. If we can get him to a hospital, he should live."

Abernathy nodded.

"You carried him back?"

"We only had one bearer team, sir."

"Right."

"They are tremendous, sir. I just wish we had more and were able to train them better."

"Train them?"

"Yes, sir."

"Doctor, I need to move on. When this is over, I want you to come and see me."

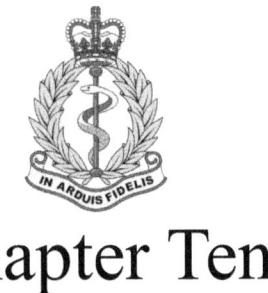

Chapter Ten

"Over one thousand were killed by the gas which attacks the respiratory system."

2nd Battalion Bivouac
South of Neuve Chapelle
13 March 1915

Despite the initial success, three days later the situation was very much as it had begun. A successful attack by the Indian division had not been followed up and our artillery exhausted its supply of shells.

In so many ways we were still learning. But that would not be clear to us for some time to come.

"Sit down, doctor."

Reporting to Colonel Abernathy as directed. I was enjoying the warmth of his tent, a cold front having blown in off the sea.

"Having a medical officer retrieving wounded from the battlefield is a bit unheard of, would you agree?"

"Sir, I think a medical officer has to do what is necessary to help his patients. I knew our men were out there and someone had to take charge."

Abernathy lit a pipe and looked at me through the haze of a very pleasant smoke.

"David, I will never admonish my officers for showing initiative and bravery. It is what this regiment has done since 1777. I would only ask that you weigh the risks the battalion is taking in losing a highly trained medical officer any time you venture onto the battlefield."

"Yes, sir. I will."

"Now, tell me what you meant by training the bearers?"

"Sir, there is another subject I must relate to you."

He blew out the fragrant smoke."

"Very well."

I related my saga with Private Ryan Jones. My focus was on the remarkable job he had done helping me care for patients. I discussed our training program and that I felt he would easily qualify as a medical orderly."

"And he was a dispatch rider?"

"Yes, sir."

"Does he still have his motorcycle?"

"No sir, it was destroyed in an artillery barrage."

"Perhaps God's retribution, Doctor McFadden."

"Quite possibly, sir."

"Let me consider what can be done. Now about this training."

"Colonel, these bearer teams are the first contact our men have when they've been wounded. Often times quick aid can make the difference from a nasty wound to a dead soldier. From what I've seen these teams are becoming experienced and taking their job very seriously. I want them to have every advantage in the field. That even means knowing who can be saved and who can't."

Abernathy sat quietly for a moment.

"Doctor, please let Major Ashcroft know I would like our bearers to receive additional training on casualty care."

I was most surprised that Major Ashcroft thought training the stretcher bearers was a splendid idea. He also placed me in charge of it, which suited me fine.

Using Jonesy and Jimmy Chesney as assistants, we set up training sessions during the long lull following what had become known as the Battle of Neuve Chapelle. We went through subjects including: casualty evaluation, field wound dressing, administering of medication and safe transport, among others. We were fortunate that Corporal Timmons attached himself to our training staff. He proved to be a talented teacher and our quality of instruction benefited greatly.

Chaplain Gallagher became a regular attendee, continuing to expand his medical knowledge. Something told me that we would find him out with the bearer teams on our next big push,

During this period, we began to receive black veil respirators. These rather cumbersome pieces of protective equipment were developed in response to the use of chlorine gas by the Germans at Ypres in April. Over one thousand were killed by the gas which attacks the respiratory system. I fear this is just the beginning to what this new concept of all out war will bring. The use of indiscriminate weapons that can affect non combatants can only lead each side to develop more lethal weapons. Where it will end is a subject I dread contemplating.

James told me he heard we were preparing our own chlorine gas for use on the Germans. Why gas bothered me so much I don't know. Perhaps the idea of destroying the lungs of a living person was past inhuman. Reports from Ypres described men who choked to death as their lungs filled with fluid. The gas also caused burns to the skin, temporary and permanent blindness in addition to chronic shortness of breath. Would there ever be an end to the science of killing men more efficiently?

Finishing a daily training session, I was helping Jonesy gather up material from our discussion of "making do" in the field when the proper equipment or medication was not available.

"Tell me about Jimmy Chesney, he seems like such a good soldier, to say nothing of the fact he is likely the strongest man I have ever seen."

"He grew up a navvy, working on the railroads. Digging tunnels, carrying rails, hard damned work."

"As I watch him around the bearers, he is a natural leader."

"Aye, that he is. But not a bully. He does more than any of his men, so they try to keep up. A good lad."

"We can put all of this equipment into my dugout," I said looking at our gear.

Jonesy broke out into a deep hacking cough.

He cleared his throat and said, "All right."

"When did you start coughing like that?"

"Last night. Had trouble sleeping, kept waking me up."

I noticed he did look flushed.

"Here, let me feel your forehead."

There was no doubt he had a fever. With the lull between actions, more soldiers had been coming down with respiratory problems.

Ten minutes later I confirmed his temperature at 103 degrees.

"You don't feel very good, do you?"

He shook his head.

"Let's get you laying down and catch this catarrh early before it gets worse." It was my earnest hope Ryan simply had a spot of a passing cough and congestion. But the high temperature would not let me push influenza out of my mind and that could prove fatal. My experience told me a young man in good health like Ryan should not be in danger, but each case was different.

So far, the Second Battalion had avoided any significant maladies that were so common amongst the army, such as dysentery and typhoid. But as Major Ashcroft had told me when we discussed camp hygiene, he had seen those diseases break out in quick order and lay a unit on its back.

The next morning, Ryan was no better. He was suffering from aches and a headache to add to his coughing. I asked Corporal Timmons to administer a steam inhalation treatment.

"Please add thyme and sage to the water, corporal. I've had good luck with that in the past. Also, I want you to be watchful for any shortness of breath. Aspirin for the headache is fine and let me know if they are effective."

Timmons looked at me with a knowing glance. He likely suspected the flu was a possibility also.

Father Mike heard of Ryan's illness and showed up with a large pot of broth which the cooks had made up under his direction. The health elixir was made up of bully beef cooked down, mixed with finely diced potatoes, a great deal of garlic and local nettles. Once well cooked, the mixture was mashed well to produce a thick consistency. It smelled wonderful.

He also produced a bottle of elderberry syrup, which I had used myself in London. Hopefully our efforts will speed Ryan on the road to recovery.

Two days after being put to bed, his fever broke. The next day I was confident he had just had a rough cold, not the flu. I administered my final medication, a hot cup of coffee, well laced with Jamesons. The smile told me I had my assistant back for duty.

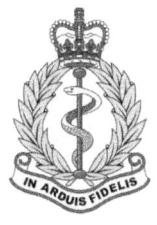

Chapter Eleven

"Our boys advanced into withering fire from German machine guns."

2nd Battalion Bivouac
North of Auchel
15 May 1915

As the battalion repositioned from our previous camp, rumors began to flow on what was in store for the Highland Light. It was clear to anyone more artillery had been deployed behind the infantry and the stockpiles of shells would allow a barrage that would eclipse anything we had ever seen. During the last several months, the losses from Neuve Chapelle had been made up by the arrival of several hundred of new recruits from the Maryhill Barracks in Glasgow. I recognized the new men, who were not only clean and proper, but also so young. Their eyes gave them away, the earnest looks and wide-open surprise as the reality of the front hit them.

My challenge was to integrate the new stretcher bearers into our now well-trained crews. Thank the Lord, I had a number of key men who demonstrated the knowledge and leadership that would let them take these new ones and break them into the brutal world of casualty recovery. We broke up Jimmy Chesney's crew, making each man a crew leader, I was very pleased when Jimmy was promoted to corporal, giving the stretcher bearers a level of recognition that had been sorely wanting.

The buildup was clearly in preparation for a major attack which we were told would open the front, allowing a major thrust forward for the BEF and the French 10th Army. Perhaps this would be the key for the final push into Germany and the end of this horrific conflict. Ammunition and significant supplies arrived to confirm we were preparing for a major attack.

"Have you seen the objective?"

James sipped his coffee. We both sat in the battalion aid station.

I nodded.

"At least 300 yards to the first German trenches."

"Good Lord, what do they expect these boys to do against machine guns."

Having seen the results at Neuve Chapelle I said nothing.

"David, this is insanity. How can we win a war when our men are mowed down like corn stalks at harvest," James added.

I had no answer. It seemed like we were going to repeat what had not worked before. Some of the officers had opined that a massive artillery barrage would destroy all of the German wire and their trenches, allowing our lads to push through to the stated objectives. We will see.

Father Mike walked up as we waited for our teams.

"Top of the morning, gentlemen."

His infectious grin made me smile despite the pit in my stomach. I was a religious man, having been raised in the church and understood the teachings and history. As a physician, I had to feel that only a supreme entity had created the human form and the wonder of life. But I found myself confused at the absurd loss of life I had witnessed in the last eight months.

"Are you ready for our lads to take their final journey today, padre?"

Gallagher turned on me.

"David, I hope that is not the case."

"Father, we both know what is going to happen."

He looked at me, but said nothing.

"Enough," James said. "We'll have enough problems today."

"Gentlemen, I'm here to offer my assistance. That's all I can do."

"I'm sorry," I said. "I guess the horror we are about to see gets harder and harder to watch."

"David, there is nothing I can say. I can only try my best to help our soldiers. Nothing else matters," the padre said.

"Then let's head out and see who we can save."

Despite a three-hour barrage, which used 100,000 shells, the German wire and trenches survived. Our boys advanced into a withering fire from the German machine guns. The results exceeded any previous losses in a very short order.

Within a hour of commencing our attack, our aid station had twenty-eight wounded, six already dead and many more still on the field according to the bearers. Two assaults had already been launched against the Germans and a third was forming up.

To add to the hell of the Maxim guns, the Germans were now using what they called "Minenwerfers" or mine throwers. These were small artillery type tubes that could send explosive shells easily across No Man's Land. Now they were using them to make the area between our trenches and theirs a killing ground. Retrieving the wounded now became even more dangerous as the smaller artillery shells were harder to hear and take cover from.

I closed the private's eyes, his wound had not been catastrophic, only a machine gun round in high thigh. But in the course of getting off the battlefield, his femur which had been broken by the bullet, sliced into his femoral artery. He died from lose of blood as he arrived at the aid station. My frustration was supreme. Our bearer crews knew how and when to apply a tourniquet. But if the wound wasn't bleeding when they start the carry, only a very observant crew would spot it as they dodge shells and machine gun fire.

Moving to the next man, I saw his eyes were open and his head turning letting me know I might have a chance to save this one, as I knelt down I saw another thigh would, but no evidence of major blood loss.

"What's your name, son?

"Glen, Glen Eakins, private," he eased out, his voice strained with pain. Through clenched teeth he slowly said, "Christ, it fucking hurts."

Pulling back his tunic I saw that the thigh wound sliced up into his groin. His testicles were severely damaged, I couldn't imagine the pain. Morphine and a bandage took care of the bleeding for now, but the potential for further hemorrhaging was high. He needed surgery, but there was no time.

Seeing Private Golden's crew setting down a stretcher I called him over.

"I need this patient back to battalion as soon as possible."

"All right, doc. Hey lads, over here."

"Private Golden, what's your first name?"

"Cedric, sir. Me father's name, I'm a junior."

"Well, Cedric junior, good luck."

I knew he would only be passed through battalion, but I hoped he would find a surgeon at the Casualty Clearing Station. His survival might very well be determined by the workload or experience of the CCS surgeons. I wished him good luck.

A soldier was helped into the dugout by Father Mike. A bandage was secured over his left eye and dried blood covered his face, neck and tunic.

"Doctor, would you take a look at Private Sullivan," the padre asked.

"Right over here, Sullivan."

The young man seemed unsteady on his feet, his one eye bloodshot.

"Here, let me take a look at this," I said as I unwrapped the bandage. Dried blood stuck the bandage to his cheek and I gently pulled it off. A smaller square pad was underneath the larger bandage, and I carefully removed it, trying not to disturb the periorbital area. His left eye and lid were mostly destroyed. I could see a severe tear over the sinus area which must have been made by a piece of shrapnel flying across his face. Part of the metal shard must have taken out his eye.

"We'll take it from here, padre,"

Working through the day, the flow of wounded never seemed to slow. It was clear the bearer teams were exhausted as the sun began to set. Our system of having Corporal Timmons examine each man first, then letting either Jonesy or I know who we should look at worked well. As medical orderlies, they both knew how to evaluate a patient, made initial treatments then bandage and finally fill out the patient ticket.

By sundown, we had seen fifty-six men, Our supplies were running low and it was clear to me the stretcher bearers had little or no capacity left to haul more bodies across the rough terrain.

Father Mike had been in and out of our station all day as he rotated from the trenches to James's station and then over to us. He came by himself out of the dark as we were finishing with our last two patients,

"Hello, padre. Come in and sit down," I said, about to offer him tea, I realized he was limping.

"Thank you, David."

"Are you hurt?"

"My left leg," he answered.

By the light of an alcohol lamp, I saw three wounds on the side of his leg, blood stained his uniform,

"Here, let me look at that."

I confirmed shrapnel was the cause of his wounds, three entry points with no exit. Two were small wounds, but the third ran for three inches across his thigh.

Probing the wounds I was able to remove the metal fragments from the two smaller wounds. It was clear the larger piece would require minor surgery.

"I'm going to bandage all three wounds, padre. The thigh will require a procedure to remove it. I'll take care of it back at camp. We're getting ready to pull out and you can go back with us. Do you think you can walk?"

"I should think so, just need to take my time."

Normally several canes were part of our pack up for this very reason, but they had been given out earlier.

"We'll give you a hand. Now, take these morphine tablets."

One of our bearers was a big strapping fella named Tisdale. He volunteered to help the padre.

Our return was painfully slow, but in time we were back at camp.

"Father, I know you are exhausted, but the sooner we remove that last piece of shrapnel the better all around."

"David, I'm in your hands, just tell me what to do."

Jonesy helped the padre remove his trousers then recleaned and bandaged the two smaller wounds.

I had a chance to examine his leg in the procedure tent under a number of lanterns. The wound was clean and I could see no fabric shreds.

"I'm going to give you some more morphine, padre. We'll give it ten minutes to take effect then I can go to work. You just lay back and take it easy."

I watched our chaplain cross himself, then relax totally.

After removing the metal fragment, we carried the padre to his dugout and put him to bed. He would need to stay off the leg for a day or so, then get used to using a cane. But if I knew him as well as I think I did, he would be back on the battlefield in no time at all.

"Ryan, can you find Corporal Timmons and bring him to my dugout?

"Right."

The day had been the toughest I had seen since arriving in France. If James saw the same number of wounded as we did, that would mean that one out of every nine men had been wounded, not counting any still in No Man's Land or on the piles of dead that always accumulated near the trenches after a major attack. How many days of battle like this before the battalion ceased to exist?

"You wanted to see me doctor?"

"Come in you two,"

I took out a bottle of Jameson's and poured drinks into three tin mugs. Handing them out to the corporal and Jonesy, I raised my cup.

"To a job well done today."

We all drank in silence.

"Corey, where are you from?"

"Glasgow, born and raised."

"What did you do before the war?"

He laughed.

"I worked in me father's apothecary shop."

"Well, it helped make you a truly gifted medical orderly."

The corporal looked slightly embarrassed and took a quick drink.

"The truth is the two of you are as good as they come. I'd put our care up against any in the BEF."

My two able assistants both nodded and I saw them grin at each other.

My father told me the only thing he truly missed from the army was the people. Now I know what he meant.

Two days later I found Chaplain Gallagher sitting on a camp stool outside his dugout. The day was mild and he seemed to be meditating with his eyes closed.

Quietly I said, "Padre?"

His eyes opened slowly and he turned to look at me. A smile appeared and he beckoned me to sit on the wooden crate next to his chair.

"David, good morning."

"You look well, I trust your pain is lessening?"

"Remarkably so. I was very lucky to have a slight wound treated by a superb doctor."

"I thank you, sir. How is it when you put weight on it?"

"With the support from a cane it is quite bearable."

"Just don't over do it."

"Yes, doctor, I will comply with your orders."

We sat for a moment listening to the sounds of the camp, a collection of voices, equipment, animals and weather. After so long, it seemed quite normal.

"Padre, do you ever ask yourself how a benevolent God could allow this slaughter to continue?"

He waited a moment then said, "I wouldn't be a normal man if I didn't."

"And what was the answer?"

"I don't have the wisdom to answer the question. All I can do is continue to minister to God's children. None of us can know the path God has decided upon, for countries or people. We can simply do our duty and trust in him to resolve the future."

It seemed a simple answer. Rather than trying to delve into the why, simply push forward with the how.

"Thank you, padre."

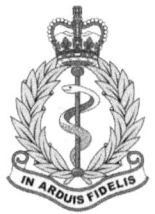

Chapter Twelve

"The gas clouds cut down the visibility significantly."

2nd Battalion Bivouac
Southwest of Loos
24 September 1915

"We will attack in conjunction with the French who will be on our right. The intent is to reduce a salient projecting into our lines from which the Germans could conduct a breakout."
Colonel Abernathy was frank with us at the meeting.

"This is not the best ground on which to conduct an attack. Jerry has the high ground which runs from Loos to Englos, which is our initial objective. In the area, the distance from our trenches to the German's main trench is over 800 yards."

The battalion medical staff, including doctors and orderlies listened as Major Ashcroft passed along the information on tomorrow's attack. He had been at the battalion officer's meeting in preparation for the attack.

"The initial attack will be signaled sometime around five o'clock. The lack of significant artillery shells will be balanced by our use of gas prior to our attack. Because of that, our men will be wearing the new masks we have been receiving over the last month. This will add to our challenge. We know the effect of chlorine gas after the German's use earlier this year. Be prepared as gas can be very unpredictable as can the reaction to men in a gas attack. I want all of you to carry your masks and be ready to use them. Once the gas is released, the wind can change. Be prepared."

The preparation for gas included the posting of a Sergeant Sedgley who had trained in St. Omer. The result of the push for some type of protection from German chlorine attacks was the "Hypo Helmet." A flannel hood, with several layers and a viewing port was soaked in a solution of sodium thiosulfate, glycerin and sodium carbonate. Breathing through the material provided a cancellation of the harsh effects of chlorine. The challenge was that each helmet had to be soaked prior to use. That process was put under the control of the battalion medical staff. Vats of the solution were placed near each muster point and the helmets were soaked. Ideally, they were soaked just prior to use, or if not, sealed in a bag to maintain the moistness.

Today, we knew when the gas was going to be deployed and the soaking could be scheduled. What was supposed to happen when the Germans surprised us wasn't discussed.

Up at 3;00 am, we moved forward to the muster points to supervise the soaking. I saw the men carrying the gas cannisters moving up to the forward trenches. It struck me the winds were light at this point. How was the gas going to spread to the German trenches if the wind didn't pick up. Without massed artillery to drive the Germans from their trenches, we were counting on the gas. Surely the attack would be delayed for favorable winds?

As expected, the men were making nervous comments as they lined up to soak their helmets. The German attack at Ypres was well known by the men. Unfortunately, as in all military organizations, the truth is often a major variation of what actually happened. We had tried to educate the battalion about what did happen in April. The lack of any defensive equipment meant the unprepared allied troops lost over 5,000 killed and wounded. The equipment was now available to protect our men from chlorine. A question unanswered was what would we do if the enemy introduced another type of gas. But for now, we should be ready.

The assault troops were equipped and mustered by half past 4:00 to begin the waiting game. Our aid station was manned with one additional member.

Father Mike, now fully recovered from his wounds, sat with us as we waited for the order to attack. He carried a cane, although he didn't need it. The cane seemed to give him a rather jaunty attitude as he scrambled around the trenches. It was clear to me the men enjoyed his ministry. They say you won't find a heathen in a trench and the chaplains of the BEF found a very receptive audience.

The first artillery salvos screamed overhead, making us all duck involuntarily. At some point I assume the signal will be given to open the gas cylinders to release the chlorine. Our men would all be wearing their hypo helmets prior to the release of the gas. The battalion would wait for the greenish gas to travel over No Man's Land, which is almost a half of a mile across. As soon as the artillery ceases, the troops will be given the order to attack, assuming the gas has reached the German lines. I thought about the men trying to see through the celluloid eye openings as they tried to negotiate rough terrain coupled with wire barriers. What we ask our men to do.

The bearer team led by Cedric Golden came into the shelter wearing their gas masks. He pulled off his flannel helmet.

"The wind has shifted. The gas is blowing back into our trenches," he blurted out, taking a deep breath. "These blessed things are bleedin' awful."

This will be a damned mess, I thought.

"I'm going up to see what's happening," I said, grabbing my mask.

The sun was now well up and in the distance past our trenches I could see an unusual haze. The sun angle coupled with the gas clouds cut down the visibility significantly. Rushing up, I expected to see pandemonium, but I realized the air was clear over our trenches. To the north, there were greenish yellow shades over friendly trenches. Were we going to be spared this time?

The air was shattered by two quick explosions just to the front of our trenches. The Boche were replying with mortars to our gas.

Running forward, I knew reaching the trench was my best chance to find cover quickly.

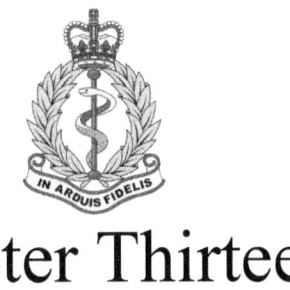

Chapter Thirteen

"Doc, what's your name?"

Southwest of Loos
24 September 1915

I felt everything around me was disturbed. The noise seemed strange and I wasn't sure exactly where I was. Then I began to understand, I was hurt. My face stung and on my left side radiated pain down my leg. Dirt was in my mouth and both eyes stung. What was wrong? As I tried to turn my head, excruciating pain took my breath away, leaving me face on the dirt trying to control my breathing.

My head felt as if it would come apart from the pain. Never have I felt such a deep throbbing pain gripping my forehead and temples. I tried to move my arms to get on my feet and knew it was futile to try. Several deep breathes helped me take measure of my situation, which was laying on my right side, face down in the side of a hill. What should I do?

Time told me to rest. Let the noise and violence pass me by, I needed to rest. Closing my eyes, I tried to block out the piercing pain in my head. It had to go away, it had to.

Voices came from behind me, muffled then loud.

"Over here."

"Right."

"Oh, Christ."

I felt hands on my shoulders slowly turning me over.

Faces looked down at me, everyone talking.

"Doc, doc, here you are."

The voice sounded concerned. I know that voice."

"Easy there, slide it down here."

"Watch his leg."

"Ches, where's he hit?"

"Wait a minute, damn you."

"His whole side, crimy. Give me a bandage roll."

I felt hands on my leg, a firm pressure, but no pain. My head.

"My head," I tried to say, not sure if it made sense.

"Gimme another bandage roll."

"Hang on, doc, we'll get you back."

The pain in my head began to ease slightly.

Laying on a stretcher, the journey seemed long.

The sun was too bright, and I closed my eyes. Suddenly an urge overtook me and I turned my head, as I threw up.

"Hold it, Ches."

A man wiped my face and throat with a white cloth.

"There go, doc. All clean."

"All right, let's go."

"We've got the doc," someone yelled.

Jostling down steps, I felt myself being lowered.

Again, faces looking down at me. I knew that face, but I couldn't come up with his name. He was quietly cutting off my tunic. Another man I also knew looked down.

"Take it easy, doc. Let me see what we have."

I felt hands examining my leg, then softly pushing on my side. Thinking I was going to be sick again I tried to roll on my side.

"Hold it, doc. Jonesy, morphine, right now."

Jonesy, that was his name.

"This will take away some of the pain," the other man said.

He then held my face.

"Doc, look at me."

He stared for the longest time like he was looking inside my head.

"Doc, what's your name?"

My name? I was starting to relax, must be the morphine. My name. The pain in my head was starting to ease.

"David McFadden, of course."

I closed my eyes. I would just rest.

Opening my eyes, I saw the unmistakable roof of an army tent. Painfully I turned my head and knew I was in the battalion procedure tent. Laying back, my head on a pillow, I ached.

"Hello?"

"Here, doc."

Corey Timmons looked down at me with a smile on his face.

"How are you feeling?"

"I've felt better, truth be known. What's wrong with me?"

He looked around,

"Doctor Ashcroft and Doctor Edwards are gone."

"Corey, tell me what's wrong?"

"Yes, sir." Shrapnel in your left leg. A pretty deep wound in your back. Part of your left ear is missing and there's a long cut on your left cheek. It also seems your head took a hell of a beating from that shell exploding."

Trying to be clinical, it seemed nothing was serious. My spirits brightened.

Corey continued, "You weren't yourself last night when they brought you in. Doctor Edwards recommended to Major Ashcroft not to evacuate you until this morning, to see if there was any improvement."

"Where's Doctor Edwards?"

"At his aid station. Major Ashcroft took over your aid station with Jonesy. The attack is continuing."

My head began to throb.

"Who's handling patient evacuation?"

"Sergeant Loefler and me."

Both very good medical orderlies, but perhaps having me to consult would make their jobs easier. I want no part of being sent to a casualty clearing station or hospital.

Sitting in a straight-backed chair with my feet resting on a wooden box, wrapped in several blankets and my head supported by a pillow I was ready to offer my assistance. The plan was to have the litters brought into the procedure tent and I would monitor, while the orderlies conducted their exam and determination of what might be done here or if the man should be evacuated. Seemed simple enough. I had taken a double dose of aspirin for the pain.

I asked the cooks to prepare hot broth to give the men coming in from the battle. It would help fight off shock and provide liquid.

The first several patients were very straight forward, gunshot wounds or shrapnel injuries, none of which were life threatening. I had them keep one man here, the other two would be going north, eventually to Rouen or Le Havre.

As the morning wore on, I was able to move over to the litters, with assistance, in order to examine the wounds directly. Sergeant Loefler was particularly good in evaluating patients, while Corey Timmons seemed to hang back bit. I wrote that off to his relative inexperience compared to the sergeant.

By the noon time, I could feel the exhaustion coming on and told them I would lay down for an hour, but to call me if they had any concerns. I did have Corey give me one half of a morphine tablet to help me sleep and it worked as expected.

By sundown, the flow of wounded slowed. Two motor driven ambulances along with two horse drawn wagons had departed for the main casualty clearing station at Ouville. From there, the wounded would move by train.

Another morphine tablet helped me with the increasing pain from my leg and back. Corey changed the bandage on my back, which included some additional cleaning. He held a mirror for me to see the wound, which looked like it had been caused by a piece of shrapnel glancing off my back. It struck me that three inches to the left and my abdomen would have been torn apart. The thought chilled me and reminded me the capriciousness of battle.

Looking up from the mirror I saw Major Ashcroft in the tent opening. His uniform was dirty, and he looked totally spent. Setting a musette bag on the ground he walked over to me.

"Doctor, how are you?" he asked, sitting down on a medical crate.

"A bit mussed up certainly, but nothing that can't be taken care of in short order."

He nodded.

"What is your appraisal of your condition?"

"The only concern I have right now is the large piece of shrapnel in my lower leg. Everything else is quite straightforward."

"I understand you worked with the sergeant and the corporal here to evaluate the casualties?"

"Yes, sir. I felt up to it and another set of eyes is not a bad thing."

He chuckled.

"Indeed. We are starting to get more reports of gangrene from wounds up and down the front. I'm concerned that your leg is a prime candidate if we don't make sure it is clean and healing."

The thought had not occurred to me. I had very little experience with gangrene but knew the price the body paid once it appeared.

"What would you suggest, major?"

"We can get you to Rouen, let the surgeons there deal with your leg and then back here to recover. Or we try the surgery here. Your choice."

While I didn't want to make the journey to Rouen. I would not be taking up the time and efforts of our people. It made the most sense and the major wasn't forcing it on me.

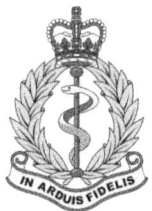

Chapter Fourteen

"...much of the trip to the hospital was a blur."

British railhead near Baileul
24 September 1915

The ambulance ride was a surprise to me in that the rough roads of rural France seemed to be directly reflected in the jolting ride. I know the driver had been instructed to hurry in order to catch the evening train, so I guess the rocky trip was to be expected.

My final contact with the battalion had been Father Mike. Returning for a foray into our most distant trenches, he had learned of my problem and returned to the bivouac. I was able to allay his concern, but he insisted that we pray together. Never one to reject a chance at heavenly intervention, I listened as he asked the Lord look over me. I felt much better as I began my journey.

In less than an hour, the ambulance arrived at the staging area. Lanterns reflected on the windows of the rail cars. Red crosses on white backgrounds were much in evidence. I saw open loading doors as teams of bearers lifted the stretchers up into the coaches.

After placing me at the end of a short queue, my ambulance crew remained nearby. I suspect they had been given some direction by the major. To work into the casualty system, I had my casualty card pinned to my tunic. This identified me, my wounds and what had been done to me at previous stations. I found myself wondering how the system would actually function, and quickly found out.

A nurse, in a long white skirt and short coat, reached down and read my card.

"Lieutenant McFadden, Highland Lights.   How are you feeling lieutenant?"

"I am doing well, nurse."

She turned to a crew of bearers.

"Take the lieutenant down to car two, please."

Car two, as it turned out, was reserved for officer wounded. In this case, I was the last stretcher to come aboard, the door closing just after I was lifted in. A second crew in the car carried me to a supporting frame which accommodated the stretcher perfectly. There were three stretchers stacked in a column, two columns running the length of the car. I was lifted to the top frame, my face only two feet from the ceiling of the car. Nurse Hayden introduced herself to me and asked if I had any immediate needs. She added the train would likely depart within twenty minutes. I needed nothing and lay back to listen as the train finished loading. I felt a quiet efficiency from the train staff. I'm sure they had made this trip many times and the process was well honed.

Without a whistle, bells or signal, I felt the train begin to move. The lights were dim in the car, and it appeared the shades on the windows were drawn closed also.

A few minutes later, Nurse Hayden returned with a cup of broth. I gratefully accepted the ceramic mug, warm to the touch.

"How long will the trip take?" I asked.

She smiled.

"That is a question I can't answer. It never takes the same time. Sometimes we are left on sidings for hours waiting for the ammunition and resupply trains coming from the coast. Other times, we go right through. I should think we will be at the hospital offload area by sunrise."

"How many casualties are on this train?"

"We are almost full, about 450 total, officer and other ranks. This latest attack at Loos has kept the trains full."

The flow of wounded in this last attack was much heavier than the battalion had seen earlier in the war. Was this a one-time situation or was the scope of battles growing as the war dragged on? A question I wasn't sure I wanted to know the answer to.

Always finding sleep easy on a train, my trip to Rouen was no different. Awakened by a nurse I didn't recognize, the trip was over and I felt rested, but very sore. The train began slowing and in ten minutes finally stopped.

As the door opened, it was clear the sun was still not up. I could hear men outside being directed to begin moving litters. In short order I was moving toward the door where lanterns illuminated the platform.

"All right, up. Move forward. Grip below."

A litter team carried me across to the far side of a wooden platform. The area around me was in darkness, but certainly there was no evidence of a town or rail station. Quite odd, but I was sure it would make sense in time.

Less than an hour later, the doors to the railcars were closed and the train released its brakes, starting to slowly move away from the platform. Looking around, there were orderlies standing around the platform and also nurses, likely from the Red Cross. But where was the hospital?

The cold was starting to have an effect. My leg began to ache. Holding my arms close to my chest, the front of my head began to ache. While I had been having off and on headaches since being wounded, this felt worse. Despite the darkness, I saw flashes of light across my field of vision.

"Here, you go," a tall nurse said as she lay an additional blanket over me.

"Would you have any aspirin? My head is pounding."

"Certainly, just a moment."

With no vehicles, motor or horse drawn in evidence, I wonder how long we'll be left here? The wind was not strong, but cold. I pulled the blanket up to my nose, hoping to shelter from the breeze.

Two aspirin might help, but as the pain increased, I wondered. Corey had told me the explosion of the shell had hit my head hard. Could there be more to it than a headache?

By the time the ambulances arrived, we had been on the platform for over two hours. By then I had moved up to morphine tablets to deal with my head pain and much of the trip to the hospital was a blur.

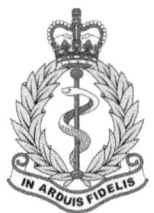

Chapter Fifteen

"The ether was harsh, but only for a short time."

Hopital Général de Rouen
25 September 1915

I opened my eyes to see I was again in some type of tent. Turning my head, I could see litter after litter on the floor of the tent, with orderlies and nurses stationed throughout. It was strangely quiet, or perhaps I was still thick headed from the morphine. The cold of the platform still seemed to be in my bones. The blanket from the morning still lay across my body and my casualty tag had been pulled out by someone.

Lifting my head, I saw a nurse several feet away and called to her.

"You are awake," she said, bending down to put her hand on my forehead.

"Where am I?"

"You're in the military annex of the Rouen General Hospital."

I knew Rouen was my destination, however this was not what I expected.

"We're admitting men as fast as we can. The number of wounded over the last several days has overwhelmed us."

She adjusted my blankets.

"Can I bring you something to drink, water or tea perhaps?"

A warm drink might go a long way toward getting warm again.

As I savored the warm liquid, I went over what she had said. I will be classified by a doctor and a course of care established. The goal was to treat all wounds and expedite release to recovery in the local area. My final question to Miss Southgate, as I learned her name, was to ask the number of casualties at the hospital. I was stunned to hear over two thousand. How in God's name can any hospital deal with a tidal wave of wounded men like that? I suddenly felt like a small piece of flotsam on a very large ocean.

"McFadden, by God it is you," a voice called.

Opening my eyes, I saw one of my closest friends from King's College, Thomas Gates.

"Thomas."

"I saw your name on a patient list and thought it might be you."

Thomas was always the life of the party, a large man whose love of life was just as big.

He looked at my casualty tag.

"It appears you are a bit banged about, eh? Didn't anyone tell you the Germans play nasty?"

I smiled.

"Quite so."

"Let's get you into prep and I can take a look."

Twenty minutes later, in another tent, Thomas conducted a very thorough exam and I felt quite comfortable I had the very best care possible. Not only a character, but he was also a superb doctor and surgeon. Both of us had been trained together and knew the level of competence of each other.

"We'll make sure the leg and back are cleaned up well, that's not the problem. I do want to take a look at your leg with the new Roentgen apparatus, before we try to remove the shrapnel. It will also confirm there's no more metal in your leg."

I had never seen this Roentgen machine operate and would welcome an introduction.

"Between Roentgen's engineering and Curie's efforts to get machines out to the armies, we've been most fortunate. I think that machine will save a great number of lives before this insanity is finished. Now, no reason to wait, let's get busy."

An hour later, a large cart was brought into the tent and shortly stopped next to my bed.

In heavily accented English, the man introduced himself, "I am operator of ze Roentgen machinery."

The cart was above my bed, but I could clearly see a large metal vessel, several supportive stands, many interconnecting wires and two large glass cylinders.

Thomas came into the tent and came directly to the machine. In short order, a wide plate was placed under my leg and one of the tubes positioned over it.

Following an admonition to remain still, the operator closed two metal switches, which were connected by cables to what looked like electrical storage batteries, much like you would see in a telegraph office. The electricity was then sent to the glass tube, which produced a humming sound.

After five minutes, he reversed his process, shutting down the apparatus.

"I will develop ze plate," the man said. Leaving the cart next to my bed, he walked away with the plate.

"Looks clear to me," Thomas said, holding the developed x-ray out to me. The large piece of shrapnel was very clearly defined, but no other foreign material appeared on the screen.

The potential of this technology was clear to me and I was now going to be able to vouch for it.

Later that afternoon, I was moved to an operating theater within the hospital. I felt quite comfortable, in a formal surgery preparing for the procedure. Despite the fact I was the patient, it was good to understand what was happening as the team got ready.

"Hello, lieutenant, I'm Glen Rossi, I'll be watching the ether today. Thomas Gates told me that you and he studied together at King's College."

"We did, he kept me on the straight and narrow."

Rossi smiled.

"Any issues with ether?"

"To be honest, I've never had it. But other than the random pieces of metal in my body, I think I'm in good health."

"Marvelous."

Thomas appeared at my side.

"You've met our resident Canadian. Don't believe a word he says and definitely don't play cards with him.

"Rubbish!" Rossi said. You Tommies just never learned the fine art of dealing."

"You've been warned, David. Now, let's get on with it, I have a date tonight in Paris."

I smiled as did Doctor Rossi as he lowered the ether cone.

The ether was harsh, but only for a short time.

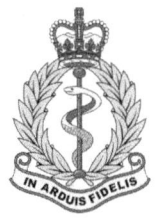

Chapter Sixteen

"...my head went light and I felt dizzy."

Hopital Général de Rouen
26 September 1915

The next morning I had a sour stomach, sore throat and pounding headache. As a tradeoff for my misery, the operation to remove the last piece of shrapnel had gone quite well and Thomas was pleased. There wasn't much he could do about the ear, other than clean it up. The injury to my cheek was straightforward. He removed the first sutures and replaced them with an attempt at the smallest scar possible.

Thomas wanted me to stay off my feet for a day to let my leg recover, then start walking with a cane. The idea of having some control over my mobility was welcome. While I tried to be a good patient, my frustration with the dependance on nurses was reaching a new high. Perhaps the theory that all doctors make poor patients was not only accurate, but more so if the doctor was young.

I saw a group of doctors entering the large tent, where I was now in recovery. My assumption was this might be the military version of rounds. It seemed to me that the heavy load of patients and limited time would not allow a great deal of retrospection following surgery. But I was a mere battalion doctor who was not versed in the ways of a large military hospital. Thomas broke away from the group and walked over to my bed.

"Finally awake, he said. "Stopped by earlier this morning, but you were still sleeping." He put his hand to the uninjured side of my face and asked, "Getting along all right?"

I nodded, but added, "Devil of a headache, stomach is upset and my throat is raw, other than that I am peaches and cream."

"Well, that sounds about right. The ether is the likely culprit, but let's see what happens with your head. The tag mentioned blast effect, you may need an extended period of recovery. That's what we have seen before when men are close to the blast and survive."

"Funny thing, I don't remember anything about getting hit. I was moving up toward a trench and then I was on the ground, not sure what way was up."

"Again, a common experience with head wounds. While you have a marvelous slash on your left jaw, I suspect the force of that explosion put an enormous stress on the brain. Liken it to getting hit in the head by Billy Wells during a prize fight. The head can only take so much."

He made sense, when I thought about being hit by the famous heavyweight boxer, I could see why I still had headaches.

"That is a wonderful analogy, doctor. But I think you need to provide some relief for your suffering friend."

"I agree. I'm going to have them bring you 30 gram codeine tablets. You know the normal dosage, but work on it yourself. Start low and build up as needed. I'll try to swing back mid-afternoon to see how it's working. No luck there, we may have to fall back on morphine temporarily."

"Thank you, Thomas."

He turned to go, then looked back.

"You know the one thing that puzzles me. If you were close enough to have cranial problems from the blast, why no ruptured ear drums?"

"Good question," was the only response I could make. Why not, indeed? When it was quiet, I had a slight ringing in my ears, but nothing of significance.

Thomas was good to his word and early afternoon found him at my bedside. With him was a very large man wearing a medical coat.

"David, I would like to introduce you to Corporal Jennings. I've asked him to work with you as you get back on your feet. In fact, we plan on doing that shortly if you feel up to it."

I noticed the corporal was holding a wooden cane with a curved top. Ready to go, clearly.

"Nice to meet you corporal," I said, extending my hand.

The big man bent down and took my hand, and nodded his head with a quiet "Sir."

James said, "Corporal Jennings was a medical orderly with the Royal Scots. He was wounded in the Battle of Mons. After his recovery, we asked him to stay on here to help with our in hospital rehabilitation.

His very pleasant face and smile did not cover up the scars on his neck, which looked quite serious. Perhaps it affected his speech.

"Glad to have your help. What's your first name, corporal?"

He looked a little surprised, but offered up another quiet one-word response, "Dan."

"Well, I'm surely ready to get up if you are ready to help."

Dan turned down the sheets and carefully lifted my legs to the floor, taking care with the bandaged left foot.

"We brought slippers," Thomas said, handing two standard issue army cloth slippers to Dan.

Once the slippers were on, Dan moved to my side, putting his left arm around my back and under my left armpit.

"Ready?" Thomas asked.

"Ready," I replied.

Dan said, "Aye."

He lifted, allowing me to lean forward and extend my legs slowly. As I straightened up, my head went light and I felt dizzy.

"You've been on your back for several days, it will take time to readjust," Thomas said as he held one of my shoulders to steady me.

The room was moving! Slowly the floor began to slant, accelerating rapidly. Dropping the cane I grabbed for Thomas, who wrapped his arms around me.

"What's wrong?" he asked.

"Dizzy…floor's moving!"

"Here, back on the bed," Thomas directed and the two of them lowered me down.

Putting both hands down on the bed, I closed my eyes. Slowly the world stabilized, and in a moment, I was able to open my eyes to a steady world.

Taking a deep breath, I said, "Vertigo, my God, that was a surprise."

"I think we need to let you settle down, then take a closer look," Thomas said.

"All right. Let me lay down. You can come back when you have some time."

As I lay there, my mind returned to my anatomy classes. If the inner ear provides the major input to the brain on orientation and movement, could the artillery blast have done something to my inner ear? Thomas already wondered about the fact that my eardrums remained intact despite my proximity to the explosion. How do I get damage to the inner ear without damaging the ear drum or canal? My jaw and my ear were hit by pieces of metal, could that have done damage without piercing the drum? But there had been the time watching the casualties at the battalion medical tent when I had been upright with no issues. At least I don't recall any issues. For the rest of my casualty journey, I was on my back the whole time. A stroke could cause vertigo, but I don't see any other symptoms. Inner ear infection? Perhaps. Meniere's disease makes no sense. The logical culprit would be some type of trauma to the inner ear from the explosion. But what?

Right after the evening meal, Thomas stopped by my bed.

"I have some invigorating tonic you might find medically warranted," he said, a grin on his face.

A quick pour into a ceramic mug told me that he had been able to maintain a stock of good scotch whiskey.

He raised his glass, "Sláinte Mhath!"

The traditional Gaelic toast to good health seemed most appropriate.

"Bit of a knocker today," he said.

I certainly felt that way.

"It has to be the inner ear," I said. "The force of the impact had some delayed effect. Or it's surfacing now. Never heard of anything like that, but what else could it be?"

"I think we try tomorrow, but go at it slowly."

That seemed like a good plan, at least it was something to try first.

"Hope I didn't scare off Corporal Jennings."

Thomas smiled.

"Not likely. What I didn't tell you today is that his wounds were easily enough to have him sent home. His speaking ability has been impaired from the injury to the larynx. He's also essentially blind in his left eye. But his attitude struck all of us and he pleaded to be able to stay and help in any way possible, not being able to return to a battalion. He won't ever give up on anybody. When he's not working with rehabbing patients, you can find him in the moribund ward sitting with the lads."

"The moribund ward?"

"That's right, you're a trench doctor, not wise in the ways of the modern military hospital."

"Go on," I said.

"The RAMC has taken on the formal process of "triage" used by the French. When a train or ambulance arrives, the wounded are screened and each casualty is directed to the most appropriate area to deal with their problem. Whether that be immediate surgery, rest to prepare for surgery, a non-surgical course of treatment, you get the idea. But it's become very clear with severity of wounds and the number of casualties, some men simply have no chance. And so, they're sent to the moribund ward, given enough morphine to deal with their pain and left to pass on. Not something the British people would like to see on the front page of the Times, but the truth all the same. The nurses do what they can. The chaplains and the other lads such as Dan spend time, talk, light cigarettes and write letters for them. When the end comes, Dan often helps with the burial, including digging the grave. He has the heart of a lion, and we're lucky to have him."

I considered what Thomas had just told me. Torn between anger over giving up on our soldiers and the growing horror of this war, I felt like I was suddenly in a horrible play. How in God's name have we come to this? I thought of my lads in the battalion. Attacking the Germans, risking horrible wounds and death, not knowing that if they arrive fighting for life at a British or French hospital, they may very well be sent out to a tent to die by the decision of one doctor. Lord God, this is wrong.

"Thomas, tomorrow I will remain upright, one way or the other. And I want Dan to take me to the moribund ward."

Thomas said nothing, he simply extended his glass to touch mine.

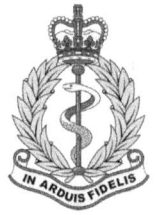

Chapter Seventeen

"Shall we visit the moribund ward?"

**Hopital Général de Rouen
27 September 1915**

"Ready?" Thomas asked.

"I am."

"Dan?"

"Aye."

The two of them were on either side of me, hands supporting my arms,

"Slowly," Thomas directed, and I began the move to the vertical at a snail's pace.

Waiting for the world to move, I was ready to fight it. The view in front of me remained stable.

Arriving at a full-sitting position I felt encouraged. Thomas looked around at me.

"Open your eyes wide and look straight ahead."

I did as he asked.

In a moment he said, "I see no indication of nystagmus."

No eyeball movement, a good sign, I thought.

"Okay, slowly move your legs over the side of the bed and sit there for a few minutes and see if anything develops."

Dan had his hand around my shoulders and helped move me to the edge of the bed.

"Thank you," I told him.

"Aye."

Putting my hands down to my side, flat on the bed, I felt a comfortable stability. Carefully, I moved my head slightly in each direction with no indications of dizziness.

"Let's check your eyes one more time," Thomas said as he stared into each pupil.

"Well?" I asked.

"Time to get on your feet, old man, slowly."

The two men helped me to rise slowly until I was standing with most of my weight on the right foot, but not entirely.

"Good so far," I said.

"Here's the cane, see if you can shift your weight."

Lowering the cane, I let the balance shift. Actually, I felt rather steady on my feet.

Walking, albeit slowly, was not difficult, but the tenderness of my left leg was quite evident.

"Shall we visit the moribund ward?"

The two said nothing, but Thomas nodded.

The official designation of the sectioned off area was "Ward D." The structure was a large multi-section tent perhaps sixty feet by forty feet. Within it there were perhaps fifty beds, with forty occupied at the moment. Several nurses were making rounds, and I saw an older man sitting at a bedside.

"That's Chaplin Beddoes," Thomas offered. "He's in here a great deal of the time. He also conducts the burial services."

I looked at Dan who was to be taking in the scene but saying nothing.

Moving slowly down the row of beds, I could see most men were sleeping or at least had their eyes closed. It was clear to me that little or no continuing care was being conducted other than what I suspected was the dispensing of morphine.

Small bags of what I assumed were personal effects hung at the head of each occupied bed. The name and number of the man identified its owner.

Thomas saw me looking at the nearest man's bag.

"We're very careful to track the personal effects of the men, including any letters or pictures they're carrying. The chaplains attempt to return them to each family.

The hero returning to the hearth, I thought, the contents of a canvas bag all the family would receive. How many little canvas bags would cross the Channel before this war was over?

I was determined to walk by each bed. While my leg was getting more uncomfortable, it was important that I saw each of these men waiting to depart the only world they knew. While they reflected the terrible damage their bodies had suffered, it was still evident they were so young.

My steady supports were quiet, letting me watch and slowly move down each row. As we finished walking down the last line of beds, I saw a young nurse carefully arranging the sheet and blanket of a man who was asleep or unconscious. She did it with such care and attention, you would have thought this was a fine hotel. She nodded slightly when she saw us and for moment I thought I knew her. But then all the nurses wore the same long gray dresses with a white apron. One more of the many nurses we so desperately needed to take care of the enormous number of wounded. And the macabre play continues.

In the early afternoon, I found myself reflecting on what I had seen that morning in Ward D. So many thoughts were wandering around my head, crossing from medical observations to the utter futility of war.

"Doctor McFadden."

I looked up to see the nurse from the moribund war this morning.

"Yes, hello."

"I saw you this morning and wanted to come by."

Strange, I thought, but why did she want to see me?

"I am glad you did," I said, not really sure what else to say.

She smiled.

"You don't remember me."

The most terrible phrase a lovely woman can ever utter.

"I..I'm sorry. Where did we meet?"

"I was one of the trainee nurses at King's College Hospital."

Good lord, now I recognized her. While there were many nurses in the training program I did remember Nurse Summers, Kathleen Summers, of course."

"I do remember. You assisted in many of my surgeries, Nurse Kathleen Summers."

Again she smiled , and it was a smile that made a person feel good. And yet here she was in this charnel house, dealing with the dying boys of Ward D, a world away from London and the world of the polite and clean.

"That seems like a long time ago."

"How long have you been in France?" I asked.

"I came over in January, right after finishing the course at King's College."

"Have you been here, at Rouen, long?"

"One month at Le Havre, then I was sent here."

She has seen at least two major offensives and the casualties that went with them.

"You have seen a great deal of suffering."

She nodded.

"I find Ward D very difficult to accept. But I know I'm young and inexperienced. Perhaps I will understand some day.

"There is no way to understand what is happening. As a doctor I find it goes against everything I believe. We don't have enough doctors, nurses, beds or resources to handle the waves of casualties. We should fight for the life of every soldier until the very end. How can simply shunt them aside to die?"

I think my anger came through my words and Kathleen looked surprised.

"Thank you for saying what I've been thinking and afraid to say."

Her words touched me. Here was a nurse who was dedicated to healing, repelled by the military system that our army had allowed to be put into place. I wonder what my father would say if he was here to observe the medicine being practiced? Was this the same army that he had so proudly served in his time of war?

"Perhaps being a battalion medical officer, I have a different view of priorities."

"You are on the lines?"

"Not quite, but close. The Highland Light Infantry, 2nd Battalion."

"I would think they would put a surgeon at one of the hospitals," she said.

"My father's regiment from the Boer War and it was expected."

"And you were wounded."

"Like many of my battalion,"

"How are you feeling?"

"Healing well after surgery. Still a bit of the wobbles and these damned headaches. But minor things."

She looked at her watch, pinned to her over blouse.

"I must go, my shift is starting in the operating room. Perhaps I can see you again while you are here?"

"I would like that," I said and truly meant it.

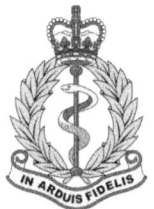

Chapter Eighteen

"And I certainly have become intrigued by Nurse Kathleen Summers."

Hopital Général de Rouen
28 September 1915

Following my morning walking session with Dan, I felt much more stable on my feet. Several times he let me walk on my own with only the cane. He stood ready to grab me, but it never became necessary. The weather had turned in a late summer warming trend and he took me outside, which was wonderful. I had not realized how accustomed I have become to living outside. The fresh air certainly helped me relax. It was wonderful being outside of the confines of tents, orderlies, doctor, smells and everything that make up the ambience of a medical warehouse.

We found a felled tree at the edge of a field just north of the hospital and sat down to enjoy the sunshine.

"Dan, you were with the Royal Scots?"

He nodded.

"In the first big fight."

"Aye."

"Thomas told me you could have gone home after being wounded."

Again, he nodded.

I wasn't sure if he would tell me, but I asked, "Why did you want to stay?"

He sat for a moment then said with a raspy voice, "To take care of the lads."

What better reason was there.

"Do you miss being with the regiment?"

He turned to look at me, and there was no need for him to say anything, his eyes told me.

Could I do that? Take Dan back with me to the 2nd? We desperately needed more orderlies. He was trained and despite his problems, would be an asset to a front-line unit. I think I might have a mission.

Kathleen Summers arrived at my bed with a small tray. There was a mug and teapot on the tray which she placed on the small side table.

"What have we here?" I asked.

"Something I believe will help you get past those headaches."

"That would be a God send. What kind of tea?"

"Feverfew. They are part of the daisy family. I have had great success with treating headaches."

She poured the steaming liquid into the mug.

"I think you will find it a pleasant aroma and taste."

Tentatively I blew on the cup and took a small sip. She was right, it reminded me of chamomile with something else.

"Thank you, that is quite good."

"I add a touch of peppermint."

As I finished the first cup and she poured a second, we talked about our lives back in England.

She was born and raised in Roslin, just south of Edinburgh. Growing up in a strict Catholic family, she attended parochial schools in Roslin, then Edinburgh. Always wanting to be a nurse, she was able to attend the

Edinburgh School of Nursing. I was very familiar with the most prestigious nursing school north of London. Her credentials were impressive already and then she trained at King's College. For a moment I thought how unique it might be to have the two of us conducting surgery after the war in the same operating theatre.

I told her of my family connection to the HLI and about my time in France. She was most interested in how we dealt with casualties on the front lines. A very unconventional lady certainly.

"I do believe the headache I think I have had for a week is gone," I said. The pain in my forehead no longer throbbed. It also appeared the ringing in my ears was better. I think I have become a believer in Feverfew tea. And I certainly have become intrigued by Nurse Kathleen Summers.

Remarkably, Thomas was able to produce replacement uniform articles which allowed me to look much more presentable only four days after my surgery. While my old trousers remained with the leg cut off from the knee to accommodate my bandages, I did have a new pair to wear when the time came to return to the battalion. With Thomas's assistance, I was able to leave the ward and bunk with him. I took my meals in the officer's mess, my RAMC insignia smoothing any questions.

"Ah, it's our battalion boy," came a voice from behind me.

Doctor Glen Rossi sat down next to me setting his food tray on the wooden plank table.

The officer's mess was a far cry from the pre-war standard. But this truly was a working mess, and no one expected anything other than acceptable food served on time.

"Good morning," I said, happy to have some company.

"All well with the leg?" he asked just before taking a large bite of fried potatoes.

"It's amazing how much better the human leg works when random pieces of metal are removed."

"Christ, the shrapnel injuries are terrible. We had one man in here with seventy-nine pieces of metal across his legs and back."

"The Germans are using a trench mortar, the *minenwerfer*. Damned thing breaks up on detonation, throwing shrapnel everywhere. At the aid station, I can deal with the life threatening bleeders, but then the wounded man is sent off to a clearing station, the hospital and the rest of the metal is still in him."

"Too bad there can't be small surgical services right at the front to take care of those things. It would save lives and keep more men from jamming up the whole system," Rossi commented, a piece of bread following the potatoes.

"Careful, you're contradicting the policy of the Royal Army Medical Corps. Do that at your peril, doctor."

Rossi snorted.

I wasn't sure I had ever heard a human make a noise like that. But then I didn't know many Canadians. Perhaps it's a North American trait.

He stood up.

"Must be off, there's ether that needs to be passed and I am the one to do it. I shall spend my war in the backwaters, never to hear a shot fired in anger. Not sure this was what I signed up for."

At the conclusion of a full hour walk, Dan Jennings and I ended up at the main entrance to the hospital. I noticed that few civilians seemed to be in evidence. Has the military assumed full use of the facility? But then France has become the battlefield of Europe, and the French people totally mobilized for the war. Would France ever be the same again?

We walked through the main building and crossed out to what I had come to think of as "tent city." I found myself moving toward Ward D, knowing that I needed to walk the beds. I'm not sure why, perhaps penance for being part of the organization that condemned them to depart this world in such a heartless way.

The ward had not changed, although I knew that some men had died while others had been added to the ward roster.

Several nurses were working the rows, and I saw Kathleen wiping the face of a man I could see had no legs. She looked up and motioned to me.

"David. I'm glad I saw you. This man is from your regiment."

I looked down at the figure, laying on his back with the flat blanket where his legs should have been.

"Jimmy," I said without thinking. It was Pomfret.

Slowly his eyes opened. They turned toward me, his head motionless. He looked at me, but made no attempt to speak.

"It's David McFadden, Jimmy."

Jimmy's eyes narrowed slightly as if he was trying to focus. Then he closed his eyes.

Automatically I reached for his medical notes, hanging next to the bed.

I saw all I needed to see. Gas gangrene had invaded his body. Attempts to arrest the infection by amputating had been too late, the deadly disease spreading upward from his legs.

"I see," I said to Kathleen.

"I'm sorry, David. You knew him well?"

"Met him on the first day I joined the battalion. Nice chap in every circumstance."

Two days later I attended the burial service for First Lieutenant James Geary Pomfret, 2nd Battalion of the Highand Light Infantry, conducted by Chaplain Beddoes.

Watching the chaplain read the burial service, I began to ask myself a question. If I had been there and was able to intervene surgically, might I have saved his life? I thought back to what Glen Rossi had said about small surgical services on the front lines. My father told me to do my duty. That duty is to save the lives of the men of my regiment. Has time come for me to draw a line in the sand?

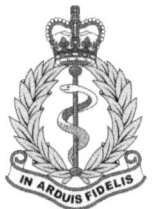

Chapter Nineteen

"Gangrene, blood loss and shock do not get better with time."

Hopital Général de Rouen
30 September 1915

Colonel James Mulholland looked like a man who does not have enough hours in his day. His face showed the effect of little sleep, many problems and contending with a war. Thomas had been instrumental in getting me in to discuss my rather unconventional idea with him.

Expecting anything from a tongue lashing to laughter, I was quite surprised to see him look interested when I laid out my plan for a forward surgical service. Two days had given me a chance to go over the problems and solutions many times. Assistance from Glen Rossi, Thomas and Kathleen helped me anticipate objections he might have.

"Sir, I have spent a year in the front lines at a battalion aid station. Through three major battles I have seen the problems these new weapons are causing to say nothing of the increase in the numbers of casualties. Anything we can do to prevent men from filling up the casualty evacuation system is important. But just as important is the number of lives that could be saved and wounds that can be minimized if we can use surgical intervention on the scene."

"But if I have to supply the people and supplies, how does that not degrade this hospital's ability to take care of the wounded?"

"Sir, during major offenses, your staff is fully employed. But those offenses so far have come every six months. In between they are underutilized. But that is when we have a constant flow of injuries from patrols, small probes and prisoner grabs on the front lines. Many wounded would never have to leave the battalion if their wounds continue as I have seen over the last year."

A knock came from the closed door.

"Yes," the colonel called.

A beefy sergeant put his head in the door.

"Sorry to bother you, sir. Just got a letter by messenger I thought you would like to see immediately."

"Very well, let me have it sergeant. Please excuse me doctor."

He opened the letter and I reviewed the point I still wanted to make."

The colonel chuckled.

"My, the timing is impeccable. This is a letter from your Colonel Abernathy informing of your promotion to captain, effective immediately. My heartiest congratulations."

He handed me the letter.

"Thank you, sir."

"Now, let's talk specifics about your plan."

Thirty minutes later I left his office with a tentative approval which depended on the answer from the battalion. I felt Abernathy would support me. This would be a benefit to his wounded and there was no reason for him not to look at it positively. The only issue would be whether Major Ashcroft would see things my way. Would the battalion commander support his senior medical officer or support a younger officer with a new idea. So far, this war had seen many new innovations, perhaps he might look at this as one more of them. For the lad's sake, I needed to make a strong argument.

"Surely you're pulling my leg," Glen Rossi said when I told him he was approved for detached duty with the Highland Light Infantry.

"The colonel agreed to a trial, if you will. If it works, he can let the rest of the army know about it."

"The front lines?" he asked.

"You won't be in the trenches, but not far behind them. But if we can treat the wounded right there, it's a boon to everyone in the casualty chain."

"When do we go?"

I told him the schedule, which would put us back with the battalion by the end of the week.

"So, get your kit ready. Do you have a weapon?"

Rossi laughed.

"I'm a Canadian, of course I have a weapon. In fact, I have what I think is the best handgun in the world. It's a Smith and Wesson .44."

"Better than the Webley?"

"You Brits may make the best whiskey in the world, but the Americans make the best guns."

There was no doubt in my mind I had the right man for the job. Thanks be to heaven he was on our side.

Corporal Dan Jennings did not hesitate when I told him of our plan for the forward surgical team. I knew that his former experience coupled with his time at Rouen made him a perfect fit for the team. When I gave him our timetable, he immediately began procuring the equipment we would need and arranging transportation.

The one challenge would be my surgical assistant. I know that Jonesy picked up procedures very quickly, but we weren't doing real surgery. Surely I could train him or Dan for that matter. Ideally, I would like to have a surgical nurse, but I couldn't imagine the medical powers to be would allow a nurse that close to the front. Or would they?

I knew that the majority of our nurses came from Queen Alexandra's Imperial Nursing Service. But there was also a contingent from the British Red Cross. I remember seeing BRC personnel working at the front, but it was always men, not nurses. But I saw no harm in at least asking the question. But could I find a nurse that would want to go so close to the fighting?

"If you were a line officer, I would send you back to Le Havre or even England for two months of recuperative leave. Your leg is clearly still healing and susceptible to those many problems we both know can crop up with traumatic injuries."

Thomas found me with Dan Jennings, going over the supplies for the surgery.

"Thomas, the most difficult thing I will have to do is walk and stand for a time in surgery. Right now, both armies are regrouping for the next big offensive. This is the time that the forward surgical unit is needed the most. I want to be there and prove the validity of the idea."

"Your idea."

"You think that I'm doing this for personal reasons?"

"I don't know why you're doing it. You're a fine surgeon. Why not stay here and operate in a theatre that is best suited to care for patients. Instead, you're proposing surgery in some dirty trench under an artillery barrage. To what end?"

"I've been there. I know that having a surgical capability where men can be treated within hours of being wounded can make a difference. Some of your patients go days between being wounded and being treated at Rouen. Gangrene, blood loss and shock do not get better with time. You know that. Maybe this won't work. If so, at least we'll know. If we don't try, we'll never know."

I noticed that Dan had quietly left the room.

"Very well, my friend. Go with my blessing, but for heaven's sake pay attention to your own health. Any problems, you get back up here and let me see you. Agreed?"

I raised my hand in a salute.

"As you direct, sir."

Later that afternoon I found Kathleen in Ward D.

"Do you have time for a brief stroll?"

"I don't have my parasol, is that acceptable?

"As this is not Tivoli, I'm sure it won't be noticed."

A touch of late summer was still in the air and we walked to a small wooded hill just north of the hospital. Away from the wards, the fresh air and smell of Linden trees was invigorating.

"Colonel Mulholland has approved setting up a forward surgical team. I'm going to take Glen Rossi as my anesthetist and Dan Jennings to run the surgery. But I need a surgical assistant. There is one young man I have trained who might do the job, but if I had a trained surgical nurse, I would be much more comfortable."

She turned as we reached the top of the hill.

While not that high, the view was good of the hospital and Rouen.

"I would volunteer to be your assistant, but I don't know what the Red Cross would say."

"What would it take?" I asked.

"I don't know, but John will."

"Who is that?"

"He's the administrator for this area of the front. His office is in Rouen, near the train station."

John Whitcomb was not what I expected. Only in his thirties, he was the antithesis of the medical burcaucrat. Tall, slim and outgoing I immediately felt at home sitting across the table from him. After a few pleasantries, I asked him to go over the Red Cross activities in the sector, realizing I had no idea what was even available.

"Most of our people are either working as nurses or driving ambulances. We do have one civilian aid center and we hope to open more."

"I was told the Red Cross has set up first aid posts in some areas of the front."

Whitcomb said, "Not in our sector, but yes we have a number of them farther east."

"If you were to establish an aid station in this sector, would you be interested in working with a team from the RAMC?"

He smiled broadly.

"Do I understand you're making an offer?"

I told him of our surgical team plan and how the Red Cross could provide additional help in the way of orderlies and nurses,

"Where do you envision this taking place?"

"In close proximity to the Highland Light Infantry's section of the front."

"But units move on, what happens when the Highland Light is ordered elsewhere?"

"My hope is that when we can demonstrate this is a good idea, whatever new unit occupies our trenches would also want to have the capability an aid station brings."

And with that, the great experiment began.

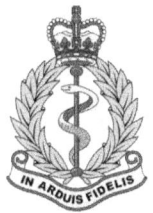

Chapter Twenty

"Sir, what I am proposing is a small surgical team."

**Second Battalion Bivouac
Near Loos
7 October 1915**

Arriving back at the battalion, my first contact was Sergeant Loeffler. He told me that James and the major were conducting a tour of the trenches and would be back by 1600. He mentioned that all of the medical orderlies were with them including Private Jones. I'd wondered about Jonesy while in hospital, but it seemed strange he was now operating on his own as a qualified orderly. Was I a bit jealous? Of course not.

"Captain McFadden, welcome back."

Major Ashcroft got up from his camp stool and offered his hand. His uniform was soiled and he looked tired.

"It's good to be back, major. The hospital at Rouen is not where I would want to spend any time, truly."

I told him about the experience being evacuated, the triage conducted at the hospital, the moribund ward and that I had seen young Pomfret before he died.

"Gas gangrene, nasty business, but what can we do, the filth and mud seem to be the problem. If a wound is complicated and also compromised by the mud and filth, you can almost be sure that gangrene is going to follow. But how do we get the wounds dealt with in a more timely manner? Can we find a better way to cleanse the wounds?"

"Sir, I think I have an answer to both of those questions.

"To gas gangrene?"

"When I was ready to leave Rouen, a courier arrived with instructions on a new procedure. It is called the Carrel-Dakin procedure. It involves use of a diluted sodium hypochlorite solution to irrigate the wound. The sooner it can be applied, the better the outcome. This also includes a surgical review to see if debridement is warranted to provide the solution the best access to the wound."

Ashcroft said nothing, clearly digesting what I had told him.

"Sir, what I'm proposing is a small surgical team that will operate in close proximity to the front, using this new method to treat wounds before the soldier is sent for evacuation. In some cases, I'm sure we can avoid evacuating at all."

"But we don't have the people for a team like that. You would be the surgeon, but what of the other medically trained assistants you would need."

I briefed him on the program that Colonel Mulholland had approved and supplied.

"Well, I'll be damned," was the major's reaction, but then he grinned at me.

"This will work, sir."

"I have every reason to believe it will. And thank God we finally have something to combat the gangrene. I think this is something we need to pass on to the battalion commander."

Following a brief to the colonel, who was very enthusiastic, I was able to search out my friends.

I found James sitting outside our dugout, his shoes and socks off, examining his bare feet.

"And what, pray tell, is your considered medical opinion," I asked most officiously.

James looked up and grinned.

"That these feet need a vacation on the south coast of England before this war goes one more bloody day."

We shook hands.

"Glad to see you are walking so well. I wasn't sure when you left here."

"Thomas Gates, a colleague from King's Hospital is a surgeon at Rouen. He took good care of me. Even used the Roentgen apparatus, a remarkable tool."

I went over my journey on the train, the triage at the hospital and the new procedure for irrigating wounds.

"So much progress in treating casualties," James commented.

"I also saw something I would have never believed. I mentioned the triage procedure, but what I didn't tell you is that some men are sent directly to a ward to die. No further effort is made to treat them other than providing them with sufficient morphine to do the job."

James said nothing for a long minute, then began to pull his socks back on.

"Good Christ, what are they thinking?"

"Everyone is overwhelmed. A train can arrive with four hundred patients. There aren't enough doctors, nurses or beds to take care of them."

"David, that's rubbish. There's always a way, it just takes men willing to do what has to be done."

He stood up,

"I believe I need a drink," he said, stepping into our dugout.

"Then I'll be able to tell you about a new idea."

The next morning Glen Rossi arrived in a French army truck. Dan Jennings rode in back with the supplies from the hospital at Rouen.

Included in the supplies were glass bottles of sodium hypochlorite which were to be diluted to make Dakin's solution. We loaded all our supplies into a dugout with a reinforced roof. Major Ashcroft was able to provide a new tent for conducting our procedures and a larger tent to serve as our ward. He contacted a squad of Royal Engineers who constructed sandbag revetments to protect both tents.

I was concerned we had no protection from aircraft attacks or more importantly artillery fire. The lieutenant from the engineers turned his men to work constructing walk down trenches with wooden roofs. This would allow us to carry stretchers down ramps into a relatively protected area in the event of attacks. This was going to be our starting layout, knowing that the nature of modern warfare would require our movement. I was sure that we could become very mobile with our truck and a system to pack up and store our material. But I needed to find another truck.

Mid-morning, Jonesy returned from the trenches where he stood watch for any casualties from the nightly patrols. Carrying two large haversacks, he saw me when coming around the main medical tent.

"Doc, you're back," he said, smiling and laying the bags at the entrance to the tent.

"You look tired, but fit," I said as he did look ten years older than the last time I had seen him.

"Up most of the night. Two of the boys were wounded on last night's patrol. The bearers are right behind me."

"Tell me about it."

"Private Russell is living a charmed life. A rifle round hit his head, putting a two inch crease in his skull. Bled like a stuck pig, but no real damage. Corporal Tway took a round in his thigh. Nothing broken, but the wound is nasty."

I decided there was no better time to get the team working.

In twenty minutes, using the main medical tent, we laid out our instruments, prepared two quarts of Dakin's solution and were ready when the bearers arrived with the two wounded soldiers. Private Russell's head wound was thoroughly cleaned, and bandaged. He would be transported to Rouen that afternoon by motor ambulance.

The corporal was exactly why this new team was in place. The wound must have been a ricochet as the damage was definitely from a tumbling bullet. His uniform was torn by the round and it was a good bet that cloth fibers, likely covered with dirt were embedded in the wound. It was time to do our job.

Glen put the corporal under and I spent twenty minutes carefully debriding the wound and ensuring there were no remnants of uniform or any areas that might conceal foreign matter. Once clean, I inserted a tube and flushed the area with Dakin's. Then I closed the wound, leaving the tube in the wound with a drain tube also.

"Let's flush the wound every two hours until the corporal departs by ambulance. Be sure to record all of this on his casualty card."

Dan acknowledged my instructions and began to wrap up the surgical area.

Glen had begun administering oxygen from a small tank via a rubber mask. This was the preferable method to bring a patient out of ether anesthesia. He told me earlier that using a mask was his choice of delivery as it concentrated the available oxygen. Bottled oxygen was in short supply at the front as it had become a prime method for treating gas victims. We could only hope the RAMC was able to expand the supply of the life-giving gas.

Suddenly an explosion ripped the morning quiet, an artillery shell landing nearby. Welcome back to the front I thought as three more shells landed at intervals north of us.

I was checking on our patients twenty minutes later when Jonesy stuck his head in the tent.

"Come quick, doc."

Outside I saw a truck with the insignia of the British Red Cross with the driver's door open and several soldiers gathering around the front of the vehicle.

Dan stood on the passenger side motioning me over.

The front windshield was shattered, with the remnant shards still protruding from the frame. Through the open door Dan was leaning over the passenger.

Pushing my way through the bystanders I saw the dark blue and white of a Red Cross nurse's uniform. Moving in I put my hand on Dan's back, and he moved out of the way. To my horror I saw it was Kathleen. Her head lay back against the seat, blood covered her face and stained the front of her uniform.

"Christ," I said softly, putting my hand on her knee.

"Kathleen, can you hear me?"

Her closed eyes slowly opened, her head turning ever so slightly toward me.

"Yes..yes."

It appeared that she had cuts across her face, done by flying glass, but thankfully I saw no puncture wounds.

"Dan, get a stretcher," I yelled.

"Kathleen, you're going to be fine, but I need to get you out of the truck."

She nodded, her eyes again closed. Looking up I saw a man in the uniform of the Red Cross, with less serious cuts across his face.

"Who are you?" I called.

"Lester Atwell, I was driving. This is Alice Bradbury, the other nurse."

A short young woman stepped beside Lester, she also wore the uniform of the Red Cross. Her eyes were wide with shock or surprise, her hand tightly clasped together.

"Nurse Bradbury, come around here and help us."

Dan had the stretcher ready with Jonesy standing next to him.

"Kathleen, I'm going to pick you up and slide you across the seat. Then we'll lay you down in a stretcher."

Her eyes opened and she looked at me.

"Thank you," she said, her voice stronger.

In a moment we had her in the stretcher. Lester, Dan, Jonesy and myself carried her into the treatment tent. My God, I thought, what have I caused?

"Kathleen, it's David McFadden."

She opened her eyes and focused on me.

"I would like some water," she said quite clearly.

After several sips of water she said, "What happened?"

"Artillery shell exploded, breaking your windshield. You have some cuts on your face that I will take care of."

"Lester?"

"Lester is fine, he helped carry you in here."

I started to clean her face with sterile water, then asked Jonesy to get me some Dakin's.

With the blood cleaned up, I found three significant wounds, her right cheek, right forehead and the left side of her head. All would need sutures.

Kathleen grimaced.

"Pain?" I asked.

"Headache, terrible headache."

The concussion from the shell, of course. That would explain her lack of awareness.

"Glen, can you get half of a morphine tablet to start?"

"Aye."

Fifteen minutes later, we gave her another half of a pill and let that work as we got the sutures ready. I also had Dan cut back her hair to get at the head wound.

Kathleen was clearly under the effect of the morphine and I began to clean and suture the wounds. This could not be a battlefield suture, not with her face involved. Using all of my skill I carefully made the smallest loops, hoping that in time the scar would be difficult to see.

Glen administered two more pills over the next hour as I went from cheek to forehead to the left side of her head. I finished with protective bandages and then let her rest.

" Lester, tell me what happened."

The young man told me they were about ten miles north of our camp when a German aircraft flew over. Twenty minutes later the shells landed near them. When he realized what had happened, he accelerated to find us. Luck had the road running into the battalion area.

He had been sent as a medical orderly and chaperone for the two nurses. His instructions were to work with them and take care of billeting and any support they needed.

"I joined the Friends Ambulance Unit in 1914, I've been in France since the start."

He was a Quaker, now I understood. The Friends as they called themselves were very active in medical support for the army. I'd just never run across any of them. Well, he seemed like a solid chap to me and that's all that was important.

"Lester, we're glad to have you."

"Just let me know what you need," he said with a most serious look on his face.

James and I vacated our dugout so that Kathleen and Alice would have quarters that were more protected than a tent. Lester's original plan had been to find a local farm or village where he could purchase accommodation. However, the German artillery activity meant than any civilian dwelling had been long abandoned. It would be up to us to house our nurses, and I decided this was a good solution for now.

An "Off Limits" sign outside our dugout was the first indication that things had changed in the billeting area. As in all military outfits, the presence of nurses was quickly known by every soldier and we saw an increased amount of foot traffic in the area. I could have sworn that I had never seen so many cleanly shaven and washed faces since arriving at the front. The only problem came from Colonel Abernathy when he learned of Kathleen being wounded.

He availed himself of a commander's prerogative and visited her the afternoon after her arrival. In the company of Major Ashcroft and myself, we announced ourselves.

Alice Bradbury opened the canvas flap and invited us to enter. The sleeping platforms had been constructed to put the occupant's feet toward the dugout opening. James and I decided that if a random shell exploded, we would rather lose our feet than our heads. It also made it easier for rescuers to pull you out.

Kathleen lay with her head slightly elevated on two of our pillows made from flour sacks. The swelling of her face was quite evident, but she was able to smile.

"Ladies, this is Lieutenant Colonel Abernathy the commanding officer of the Second Battalion. Colonel, Nurse Alice Bradbury and Nurse Kathleen Summers."

My very brave commanding officer seemed at a loss for words, a problem I had never seen before.

"Ah, very glad to make your acquaintance ladies. I am most sorry for the events of yesterday. We are well within the range of the German's long guns and never know when we might be attacked."

Alice and Kathleen said nothing but were very focused on the colonel as he continued, "It does bring up the very real danger that you both would be in if you remained with the battalion."

He paused as if searching for his words.

"Quite so," the major added quietly.

"Perhaps this was not a good idea after all," the colonel continued.

"Sir," Kathleen broke in. "Nurses go where they are needed. I am a surgical nurse and Nurse Bradbury is under my tutelage to also qualify to assist in surgeries. We are here to do our duty, just as your brave soldiers. Please do not take that away from us."

As we walked back to the colonel's tent, I was surprised and pleased that he had decided they could stay with the team. Kathleen's request, coming from someone who has been wounded and wants to stay in the fight was powerful. I was quite proud of her.

"Remarkable, quite remarkable, McFadden. This in a new world, a very new world."

"Most certainly, sir."

And it was and she was a quite remarkable woman.

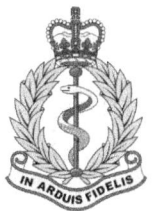

Chapter Twenty-One

"You are very perceptive, doctor."

Second Battalion Bivouac
Near Loos
15 November 1915

As winter settled over the western front, the activity by both sides decreased. While not a complete cessation of hostilities as was often the case in previous wars, it was if both armies where resting and rebuilding for the spring offensives.

For my little part of the war, I was pleased as it gave us time to truly train for what I knew was coming, Kathleen had recovered well and resumed her nursing duties only three weeks after being wounded. Nurse Alice Bradbury blended in quite well and proved herself to be a superb student. I found it quite interesting that Jonesy took great interest in passing along his knowledge to her on how to work with me. Truth be known, I believe my trusty orderly is a bit smitten.

Not one to cast the unfair stone, I also was more taken with Kathleen as time went on. Not only a superb nurse, she took the hardships and inclement weather in stride. The truth was that the decrease in patrols left us less busy than I would have liked. The occasional wounded soldier found himself at the center of a medical whirlwind. It was good to see the average Tommy getting the care only the most affluent could expect in London.

Word of our clinic spread along the trenches, and we began to treat any and all who were willing to make the trek to our tent in the woods as we called it.

I made an agreement with the quartermaster that if we received pigs, live or carcasses, we would be given time to perform surgical procedures on the departed animal. Pigs, have a remarkable similarity to the internal layout of humans. Consequently, practicing incisions, sutures, resections and projectile removal was invaluable in keeping the team in best form and ensuring Nurse Bradbury's training was exemplary.

Kathleen sipped her coffee, the steam rising off the hot liquid. The temperature in the treatment tent was almost comfortable. The cast iron stove was kept going almost continually and the tent was the normal area the team spent their time. Dan had taken it upon himself to keep the stove in the treatment tent and the ward supplied with plenty of firewood.

I poured myself a cup of coffee and sat down next to her. She had stopped wearing the bandages and her sutures had been removed. I thought the scars were as good as could be expected, but she had not mentioned it. Still pink and reddish, I knew that in time the coloration would return and hopefully the scars become less noticeable.

"Are you interested in trying to go home for Christmas?" I asked her.

"No, I don' think so. Are you?"

I shook my head no.

"The journey isn't worth it. My dad is always working and my mother died when I was 14. No siblings, so nothing really to go home to."

"She smiled. I have a wonderful family, and Christmas is always a special time."

"They why not go?"

"My family didn't want me to come to France. In fact, it was the first time I actually argued with my mother and father."

"And you don't want to go home with your wounds so recent."

"You are very perceptive, doctor."

"They will get better, you know that."

"It's funny, maybe because of where we are, they don't bother me. Perhaps at home, going to the theatre it might be different."

As she sat here, a blanket around her shoulders, scarf secured around her throat and over her head, it was hard to imagine going to the theatre.

I smiled at the thought.

"And how does Doctor McFadden react to those scars?"

The question caught me totally by surprise.

"How do I react?"

She looked very serious.

"Tell me what you think. Do they bother you? Please be honest with me."

How could I explain to her that she was Kathleen, scars didn't matter, nothing mattered.

I got up and knelt next to her. She looked at me questioningly. And I kissed her as softly as I could on her lips, then her left cheek then right.

"I love you, Kathleen Summers, no matter what."

She reached out, lightly touching my cheek.

"And I love you, dear man."

The holiday season of 1915, despite being on the front, was one of the best times I have ever had over the holidays. Every emotion was accentuated by the spirit of warmth and humanity. The smallest blessings were accepted with great appreciation and the comradery a thing of wonder.

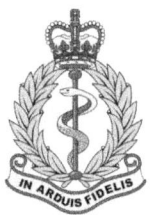

Chapter Twenty-Two

"The Germans are sending more men to the front."

Second Battalion Bivouac
Near Loos
1 March 1916

Spring of 1916 came early on the Western Front. New troops arrived from England, supplies became more plentiful, and morale improved among the men of the Highland Light Infantry.

An all-out war was declared on both lice and rats. Dogs and cats began to appear among the trenches, procured from the local villages and some even from farther away. Soon we got to know the names of the best rat hunters and cheered them on their daily forays through the trenches and dugouts.

The weather made it possible to rotate men back to the rear where they were given bathes and their clothes boiled to kill the lice and their eggs. While these were only short-term solutions, I think everyone felt better that the army was trying to deal with the lice. Not just irritating, they spread trench fever, a painful but normally not fatal malady that made the patient extremely uncomfortable.

We also saw a marked improvement in the food quality. I think the army simply took this long to figure out what it takes to supply an army that now numbered close to one and one half million men. The French also had taken time to sort out their food production in the middle of the war.

Members of the newly created Graves Registration Commission began to be seen in and around the billeting areas. Originally from the Red Cross, the organization had expanded to become an official army organization. I thought of those three men we buried that first day on the line. Would they try to find them? And then what?

As expected, the patrol frequency increased. While there were no rumors of a large offensive, the chain of command continually was testing enemy positions across No Man's Land.

Major Ashcroft had been called away to a medical conference in Rouen the last week of February. It made me think that the chain of command was beginning to put plans in place for the expected spring offensive. What better way to get ready for war than get the medical types together to plan how to patch up the casualties.

"Good news, Doctor McFadden. It seems that your idea of having an intermediate stop on the way to the casualty clearing stations had caught on. In fact, the RAMC is now establishing what they will call Regimental Aid Posts across the front. Your trial period seems to have become a fact of life. Congratulations."

"Thank you, sir. I'm glad things worked out."

"In addition, you have been promoted to captain and will relieve me as the battalion medical officer."

I was stunned. It seemed to me that I was still the "new boy" and only getting my feet on the ground.

"Major, what about Doctor Edwards?"

"Captain also, but you will have the supervisory job. If the system works correctly, another doctor will be assigned to the battalion. I'll be going to the division staff as the senior medical officer. My job will be to make sure the battalions and regiments have what they need to get the job done."

"Congratulations, sir. With your battle experience, no one is better qualified to provide support to the field teams."

I really felt the major would be a good man to have at headquarters. He knew what it was like down here and had shown me he had the backbone to get the job done.

"Mon capitaine, I hear congratulations are in order."

I turned to see Father Mike with a full parade ground salute and big grin on his face.

"Just a good protestant trying to do his job, padre."

He offered me his hand and slapped me on the back.

"Glad to see it me boy, the lads are in good hands."

"I think this year is going to be a tough one from what I'm hearing. The Germans are sending more troops to the front and that can only mean an offensive is coming.

The chaplain's face turned serious.

"A terrible thing war is and never to be forgotten."

"Perhaps you might join me in a friendly libation to celebrate my August appointment."

"Most certainly, I consider that an order from a superior officer."

The major left the next day right after the colonel signed the paperwork for our promotions. I was concerned that my friend might find it hard to be officially working for me, but that was soon put to rest. He took me aside, shook my hand and let me know that he thought I was the man for the job. I was a fortunate man to have friend like James Edwards. It was one of the few things that made this war bearable.

A long walk by myself gave me time to consider what I needed to do. The medical department of the battalion was experienced and dedicated. Keeping them supplied was important as was training any new members that might be assigned. Was there a way to step up our bearer training with Corporal Chesney?

The next day I was getting ready to review the supply status when Sergeant Loeffler walked up with a young officer and another sergeant. I immediately saw the RAMC insignia on the lieutenant and suspected he was our new doctor.

"Captain, this is Doctor Bernard, just reporting in to the battalion for duty."

He looked to be in his mid twenties and I suspect he was recently out of medical school. He was quite thin and his new uniform seemed to hang a bit on him.

Doctor Bernard saluted and I stood up, offering my hand.

"Welcome to the Highland Lights, doctor, we are very glad to have you."

"Thank you, sir."

I looked toward the new sergeant and Sergeant Loeffler spoke up.

"This is my relief sir, Sergeant Nance. I will be joining Major Ashcroft at division."

Nance was a sturdy looking sort with a pleasant face and short cropped hair. He saluted and I shook hands with him.

"Sergeant Loeffler, why don't you get them settled. I'll plan on meeting with each of you this afternoon."

Doctor Randall Bernard was indeed a new graduate of the University of Liverpool School of Medicine and the RAMC training program. I took about an hour to go over lessons I had learned over the last year and a half. I told him Corporal Timmons would be his medical orderly and explained our normal deployment during assaults.

"We are pretty informal in our group. Feel free to call me David. What do you prefer?"

"My friends call me Rand."

"Rand it is."

"Sir, eh David, there is something you should know."

"Go ahead."

"Well, I am engaged. I was supposed to join Mary's father's practice in Liverpool, then I was conscripted."

"So, you didn't volunteer?"

"No, sir."

I knew the Military Service Act of 1916 opened the conscription to meet the needs of the war. But I didn't think about doctors.

"I guess we need to talk about that. Up until now, this has been an army of volunteers. Now with a new input, I am sure things will be different. As I went over what we have learned with you, I suspect you understood this is a very brutal challenge for a doctor in a forward aid station."

"Yes, sir."

"Can I count on you to give it your best?"

"Yes, sir. I will. I am just afraid how I will react."

"I can't lie to you, the wounds can be horrific. But these are our lads and they are counting on us to take care of them. You will find they are the best in the world. They put up with terrible conditions, disease, poor food and machine gun fire. But they fight and persevere. I have the greatest respect for these men, I think you would also."

He nodded, but his eyes told me that he wasn't sure.

"I better go and get settled in, sir eh, David."

Sergeant William Nance was a complete departure from the very proper and sedate Sergeant Loeffler. Nance had just returned from duty with the Mediterranean Expeditionary Force and eight months on the Gallipoli Peninsula. There was something about him that I could only call rugged. He was relatively soft spoken, but there was an underlying hardness. He like his predecessor was a career army man, having joined up in 1906. When I talked about his medical history, he had been involved in skirmishes with natives during his time in India. Qualified as a medical orderly, he also was an anesthetist having spent time at the Royal Medical Hospital in Netley.

"We have been using two forward aid stations with a doctor and orderly at each. The stretcher bearers rotate as needed."

"If you have no objections, I think my place is at the forward positions."

Quite a change from Sergeant Loeffler, who always remained at the rear. But I liked his desire to be on the scene. I went on to describe our regimental aid post and the surgical capability.

"Good idea, and can I ask you to remain close to Doctor Bernard. He is new to the front and I think he is in for a big shock."

"Understood, sir."

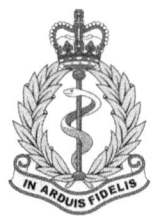

Chapter Twenty-Three

"Will these guns ever stop?"

Second Battalion Bivouac
Near Albert, France
30 June 1916

The first of June, we moved from our long-time location near Loos to a new area near Albert. Only twenty-five miles by land, we found ourselves in another world. Other units were in place before us and on arrival we learned about the upcoming offensive.

The French are under extreme pressure from the Germans at Verdun. Starting their attacks in February, the Germans have thrown twenty divisions, over one million troops, at the French. This may be their main thrust to force an end to the war this year. We'll attack in this area of the front to force the Germans to split their forces and give the French some respite.

Our battalion, now attached to the Third Division has been tasked with attacking a major German strongpoint near La Boiselle. We know there are multiple trenches backed up with significant artillery and supply dumps. I can see the company commanders are not optimistic after making reconnaissance patrols in the area.

The other major change for the battalion was the issue of the new "Brodie" helmet. The French had introduced a helmet in 1915 which provided some protection from shrapnel. Brodie designed this helmet as well to primarily provide protection from shrapnel burst above the soldiers. We would see what difference the new helmet would provide in the very near future. I dearly hoped it would live up to its expectations.

Tomorrow we will finally attack. The massive multi-day artillery barrage will cease at 0730, and over 100,000 men will attack on a 15-mile front. The Highland Lights will contribute the 950 men of our four companies. If the artillery does its job, the barbed wire will be destroyed, and our men can penetrate to the enemy trenches. Of course, the machine guns will be the greatest threat, but our artillery should take many of the gun emplacements out before our men attack.

In preparation, James and our new doctor will man the two aid stations while our team remains in the treatment area, taking care of our wounded brought in by the bearers. Thoughts of Loos ran through my mind, knowing what was coming. Dan and Kathleen had seen the results of Loos at the hospital at Rouen, but not at the front. This would test us all.

Last night four motor ambulances arrived, intended to move the wounded from our area to a casualty clearing station located about ten miles west of our position. I looked at a map and saw the CCS was expected to take the wounded from two divisions, then pass them on to the hospitals at Rouen and Étaples. From there, they would be processed to Boulogne and Le Tréport. From there, some would be sent to England. I could only hope that the system had matured from last year.

Stopping by the treatment tent, I found Jonesy going over the instrument trays. Over the last several days, we had re-sterilized our surgical tools using a solution of boiling water and carbolic acid. We were prepared to do the same tomorrow, using our cast iron stove and two large kettles. I could only hope it wouldn't be needed.

"Ryan, ready for tomorrow?"

He looked up, his face bleak.

"I'd tell ya, doc. I went down to the for'd trench to check on some of the lads and they let me see through the periscope. Criminy, the wire is the thickest I've ever seen. I don't know how our boys are supposed to make it."

"The artillery says they can blast it apart."

"Aye, 'n they said the same thing at Loos."

He was right, while the artillery officers complained of a shortage of shells, they didn't cut the wire before the attack.

Kathleen came through the tent entrance, the strain apparent on her face.

"Will these guns every stop?"

"Not until tomorrow," I told her.

She sat down and said, "I never understood how it wears you down,"

I nodded, she was right, the incessant noise worked its way into your head, slowly pulling at your sanity.

"Those poor men in the trenches, waiting for tomorrow."

She understood the trial the infantrymen were undergoing. Any of them will tell you that waiting is the most difficult. Some crack at the order to attack, but most are ready to get on with it. Every man telling himself it will be the other fella that goes down, not him. But those who took part in the Battle of Loos, will know better.

The next morning, I knew I must go down to the trenches. I needed to see what the lads were being asked to do. While there was nothing I could do about it, I knew that I had to be there.

Captain Larry Anholt, commander of A Company, stood at one end of the far right battalion trench. He and I had become friendly over the last year, but not good friends. All in all, he was a fine officer, who had been with the battalion since the first day in France. I could only hope the experienced officers would make a difference during the attack. It struck me as absurd the most senior officers to actually be in the middle of the attack were the battalion commanders. All of the other senior officers were some distance away from the actual battleground. How could they understand what was happening unless they were here? Messengers can't convey the feel of the battle or problems that need fixing quickly.

"Larry."

Anholt turned to see me.

"Doc, what are you doing down here?"

"Just wanted to be here."

He nodded, taking a cigarette from his tunic pocket and lighting it from the one he was already smoking,

There was no need to try and make small talk, he was probably already in the attack or thinking those last thoughts of loved ones.

The troops seemed to be keyed up. All were standing on the wooden duckboards, their rifles at the ready. Talk among them seemed to be nonexistent. Most were staring at nothing. What struck me as different was for the first time they were all wearing the new Brodie helmet. While it did look quite odd, the potential to prevent shrapnel injures specifically was significant. I doubt it will do anything to a Mauser or Maxim bullet, but it could help.

Suddenly the ground shook and I turned to see a huge explosion of dirt and smoke several hundred yards across No Man's Land. It must have been the underground mining I had heard about. The engineers had been digging tunnels under the German positions to place explosive charges. It was fascinating to watch the dirt thrown hundreds of feet in the air, spreading around the explosive center. Whoever was on top of that has gone to meet their maker, hopefully saving a lot of our boys.

As the sound of the explosion died away, I heard the shrill whistles calling the men to the attack. There had been corridors cut in our wire, to allow our attack to proceed as quickly as possible to the enemy territory. Now the lines of men made their way toward the wire. I could see some running, others lagging behind. How do you charge an enemy line, a dead run or at a steady pace? Perhaps it depended on the man himself. It seemed to make no difference as men were falling in the front and rear of the attack. Many men were falling.

The sound of German machine guns ripped across No Man's Land. My God, the noise told me there were numerous guns now opening up on our attack lines. The men were still several hundred yards from the enemy's first trench line. It was going to be a blood bath.

I saw men going down, not sure if they were taking cover in shell craters or hit by the machine guns. The firing was non stop, giving mute evidence the bombardment did not do what was expected. How could the Germans have survived a weeklong barrage and still be putting up this kind of defence?

Down the line I could see stretcher bearers heading out toward our troops. I needed to get back to my post. I had seen too much already.

Turning, I saw Colonel Abernathy standing with his small staff behind the main trench. He held binoculars up to his eyes, as did two of the other officers. What must he be thinking?

I took the path that led back to camp and passed the group. The colonel lowered his glasses and saw me. I raised my hand in a salute. He looked at me and nodded, the look hard to discern. Was he angry or frustrated or distraught? He was watching his battalion savaged by the German machines.

A Company and half of B Company made up the first wave. Now the second wave waited for the shrill of the whistles to signal their attack. Would Abernathy send the second wave into that cauldron? The high command sitting miles behind the lines would have no idea of the slaughter taking place in No Man's Land. It was if the men of the Highland Light Infantry were damned to die because that was the plan. It was lunacy.

Five minutes later, as I continued back toward camp, I heard the whistles coming from our trenches.

The team was ready when I returned, all standing in the treatment tent. They must have sensed my shock at what I had just seen, their faces reflecting both concern and fear.

"It will be bad, very bad," was all I could say about what I had seen.

"Ryan, go out and bring in the ambulance drivers."

I told the drivers that we were going to be overwhelmed by the number of casualties. They had to let the casualty clearing station know the situation and get as many ambulances, motor or horse-drawn, down here as soon as possible. The four nodded, but I don't think they understood the magnitude of the problem.

It took an hour before the first stretchers began to arrive. The mild weather made our triage outside much easier, and I realized very quickly this was not going to be a measured response from our team. Instead, today we would focus on critical lifesaving actions. We had to count on the doctors at the CCS, the hospital transport and at the hospitals for the follow up. Our job was to provide enough care to get them to the Casualty Clearing Station alive. If we could pass them through with no action, all the better.

The first seven casualties were able to be loaded into the ambulances after examination. All of the wounds were from bullets, which I assume primarily came from the Maxim guns the Germans were firing when I left the trenches. The German machine guns and their primary rifle used the same cartridge, so it is difficult to tell unless there are multiple wounds. My thought as I examined the lads is that these are the men that were fortunate to be hit in areas that were not immediately fatal. How many of them are lying in No Man's Land dead or dying right now.

At mid-morning, Jimmy Chesney arrived with a casualty who had been shot in the chest. He was exhibiting a marked pallor, his lips almost blue and skin ashen grey. It was certain to me that he was bleeding internally and had no chance of reaching the casualty clearing station.

The team quickly put him under ether anesthesia.

"Glen, please start a drip with Ringer's right away."

I could only hope that the saline solution would help his blood pressure long enough for the operation to proceed.

I opened the wound, which was four inches below the sternum, centered on the left side. The bullet appeared to have entered directly, neither tumbling nor slashing. I hoped that would make following the path of the bullet easier. The lack of significant bleeding told me that he was in extremis. It allowed me to find the actual tear in the abdominal artery that had produced internal bleeding. The repair was straightforward, and I expedited the closure of the incision. The bullet remained lodged somewhere, and a second operation would be needed as soon as possible. But this would hopefully allow him to get by until he was able to withstand another procedure.

As the afternoon progressed, we were able to perform three operations, but primarily we adjusted dressings, re-bandaged when needed and provided medication. The problem soon became clear. There were so many wounded the ambulances were not able to keep up. One of the motor ambulances broke down and the other three took over two hours for a round trip to the CCS. We were able to use two horse drawn wagons for those with less serious wounds and a dozen casualties were able to head for the next stop.

The delay let us administer saline to many of the wounded and I began to worry if our supplies would last. Earlier we pressed Lester Atwell into service with the Red Cross Truck. While not an ambulance, it could carry four stretchers. On his third run, I put Glen Rossi with him to procure supplies from the Casualty Control Station. I hoped a lieutenant would have the ability to draw what we needed and get it back here.

The sun set and we still had forty-two wounded under our care. Our efforts had to continue through the night, but now we had to improvise with extra blankets as the temperature went down, lanterns to see what we were about and food for those men who were able to eat.

A runner told me that Rand and James were remaining at the aid stations as the bearers made continued trips into No Man's Land looking for wounded. I was sick thinking that we had seen sixty wounded off to the CCS, and still had over forty here. How many were dead and how many more laying in that hell between the trenches. It was an ongoing nightmare.

Under canvass tarps, we tried to make our men as comfortable as possible. The night was mild, and the men were mostly quiet. I watched Kathleen and Alice move among the wounded, kneeling down to check bandages, administer water and pain medication and try to keep their spirits up.

I saw a soldier I recognized and went over to check on him.

"Private Butler, how are things with ye?"

The young man turned his head to see me.

"Ah hav fel better, truly."

I took my torch and reviewed his patient tag. Two bullet wounds, left leg, minimum blood loss, nothing broken.

"They'll git the leg well, don't worry."

"Doc, have a fag?"

I reached into my tunic and pulled out a pack of Players. I lit one for him and he took a deep drag.

"Ah, better," he said.

I felt a bond to this man and all of the others. Doing their duty for their country, now in pain, perhaps disfigured or disabled for life, but their spirit was not broken. I could only do my very best for them as long as this horrific war continued.

I saw James walking up with Corporal Ennis. He dropped his haversack and sat down on one of the ammunition boxes.

"I've never seen anything like it," he said, his voice tight. "A proper cock up. The artillery barrage didn't knock out the German strongpoints and they fucking killed our boys, line after line. This is not how you win wars, sending your men into a killing zone, then doing it again. Good Christ, what are the fools at headquarters thinking?"

"Any estimates?" I asked.

James sighed.

"I don't know. Thirty percent killed or wounded?"

The number was hard to comprehend. Three hundred men from a battalion of nine hundred dead or out of the battle.

"What's this here? Why aren't these men at the CCS?"

"Broken down ambulance, too long a trip and the CCS is almost an hour away. We'll keep at it all night, but I'm sure they're totally overwhelmed as well. At least here we can take care of our lads."

"Christ," he said in disgust.

"Go get some food, have a scotch and get some sleep," I told him.

He laughed, but there was no humor in that laugh.

"We just came back for more supplies. The bearer teams are still bringing in wounded and the word is there'll be another attack at 0830 tomorrow."

James sat quietly, his gaze at his feet.

"Larry Anholt was killed in the first wave," he said quietly. "He's been here from the start. Let's get the God damned generals down here and let them lead the next attack."

I thought about our men, living with dirt, lice, disease and death while the generals ate off linen and crystal at the nearest chateau. But I guess nothing has changed for thousands of years. The general's role in war is to send other men to their deaths and then write their memoirs.

"Have you seen Rand?"

He shook his head. If the attack had this effect of James, my God what has it done to the new man?"

Kathleen walked up and said, "The colonel."

Kneeling down by one of the lads, our battalion commander was quietly talking to him. I watched him reach down and put his hand on the man's shoulder, then stand. In the shadows, I watched him move from man to man. Was he offering thanks, or comfort or hope? What can you say to men that have been fed into a slaughterhouse? But I knew Abernathy. He was old army and this had been his life. The regiment was his world, his family. I would not interrupt his time with the lads.

But he finally walked over to me and nodded.

"Sir."

He sighed. For a moment I wondered if he was all right.

"How many?" he asked.

"Two hundred and sixty have either been sent on to the CCS or still wait here."

"Christ Jesus," he said softly.

"Tomorrow, sir?"

"We'll attack at 8:30 tomorrow."

What was there to say?

"Yes, sir."

"Thank you, doctor," he said, walking toward the trench line.

Kathleen came up next to me.

Turning toward her, it seemed the most natural thing in the world to take her in my arms. We said nothing but held each other in the darkness of that terrible night.

I found Rand asleep at the edge of the laid out stretchers, Corporal Timmons sat next to him his back against a wooden trunk.

"Corey?"

He looked up.

I knelt down.

"Are you okay?"

He nodded.

"Just tired, like everyone else."

"How is Doctor Bernard."

"Ten years older than he was this morning."

Quietly I asked, "How did he do."

"He did just fine. Once the initial shock wore off, he turned to and did some good work. Sergeant Nance made a big difference, just being there."

Thank God.

"Corey, get some sleep, we need to be ready for an attack at 8:30 tomorrow."

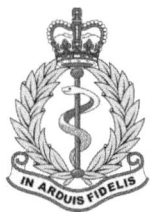

Chapter Twenty-Four

"...we lost almost five hundred dead, wounded or missing."

**England
27 June 1916**

Staring out the grimy rail car window, I watched the field of Yorkshire pass as daylight slowly slipped away. In a first-class compartment on the mid-day Caledonian Express from London to Glasgow, I kept trying to reconnect to the world outside the trenches of France. The other three passengers made small talk, but my thoughts continued to return to the last three weeks. The press called it the "Somme Offensive," as if a wave was moving forward to engulf the German invaders. Absolute drivel. The casualties continued to mount with little or no progress against the enemy.

Thank God, we lost no members of the medical staff. One team of bearers were all wounded when a minenwerfer exploded, but nothing serious.

Our battalion was being reconstructed, needing over four hundred new soldiers to get back to strength. I saw it as a chance to take leave and see my father. Truth be known, Kathleen's decision to finally go home and face her family was the real reason I decided to go also. I knew she dreaded the confrontation and wanted to be in England in the event she needed my support.

When the battalion was sent back to stand reserve and re-equip, the total number of effectives, including all staff support totaled three hundred and seventy-two. As an infantry battalion, we were more like a reinforced company.

There had been a strange quiet among the men as we moved west to the area set aside for rest and regrouping units. It was clear to me that the men were totally exhausted. But my sense was the exhaustion was a combination of the stress of combat, the shock at seeing so many mates killed and the future that could only be described as bleak. The massive effort by the BEF had produced nothing in the way of a significant breakthrough. Soldiers could only see a future of continued battles with no chance of surviving the war. Having no experience like this to compare, I could only do my best to take care of them and let the future unfold.

Our medical work had been brisk, with many of our walking wounded still with the battalion. Most of the wounds were from shrapnel along with the random dislocation or sprain. A few men were very withdrawn and seemed to be suffering from a mental aftermath of the battle. Certainly not a surprise, even if the battalion was mostly made up of experienced soldiers. What would the battalion look like with over four hundred new soldiers over the next few months?

Rand Bernard quickly adapted to a version of medicine I know he never imagined during his studies in Liverpool. He put his thoughts together when he told me, "Nothing could have ever prepared me for what I have seen in the last three weeks."

He was now a veteran.

We'd been able to take over a small farmhouse, abandoned by the owners. It allowed us to set up a treatment area. There was enough room for eight temporary beds to treat some of the men who were the most serious. It made no sense to send anyone to a Casualty Clearing Station or on to any of the nearby hospitals, all of which were overwhelmed by the number of wounded men from the first week of the battle.

The presence of Kathleen and Alice seemed to have a very positive effect on the men in our little ward and to those who came by to have their bandages changed. James had told me that the lads seemed to be quite proud of their "angels of mercy."

The warm weather also made bathing and delousing much easier. Clean clothes and full stomachs went a long way to helping the men forget the week of battle that had decimated their ranks. I don't think they will ever completely get over the pain of what happened, but they are young and that is positive.

It seemed that everyone was taken with the urge to get away and Jonesy had been able to get leave for one week. He chose to take one of the "leave trains" to Paris, having heard the tales from the men who had visited the capital. Alice had been recalled to Rouen which had been a disappointment for both. While he didn't confirm it, I believe the plan was for them to meet in Paris. It seemed there might be a spark of true love between the two. A bright spot in what had been a very dismal period recently.

Pulling into Glasgow Central Station, I checked my pocket watch, noting it was 8:14, making our arrival almost on time. With only a small bag, I was able to beat the crowd to the holding area in the front of the station. There were both motor taxis and horse drawn carriages of different types. Pushing past several hawkers, I engaged a driver.

Familiar sights, even in the darkness were comforting. The streetlights, so foreign in the battle fields of France seemed to be welcoming. With the windows in the car open, the sweet smell of Linden trees confirmed I was home. Relaxing, I took my cap off and let my mind soak in the idea of this foreign environment.

The heavy knocker on the entrance door made more noise than I remembered and I stood waiting for a response. In less than a minute I heard the bolt sliding open and the door swung open.

"Yes."

Silhouetted by the entranceway lights, Mrs. Randolph, our housekeeper stood looking into the darkness.

"Oh, my! David, it's you."

"Hello, dear."

She opened her arms, and we embraced. As a member of the household for my entire life, she served as a surrogate mother as I grew up. Now holding her, I realized how much I had missed home and hearth.

"Come in," she said, "Please. Oh, it is so good to see you."

Stepping into the light of the entryway, I laid my bag on the floor and looked around, noting that absolutely nothing had changed except there were electric lights providing illumination. When I had left for the war, gas provided all lighting in the house. The world was changing everywhere.

"Oh dear, your face," Mrs. Randolph said almost apologetically.

"It's nothing, it really isn't. Besides the ladies love it, I tell them it's a fencing scar."

She looked at me with a quizzical look, then shook her head.

"You always were incorrigible," she said taking my hand. "But I am so glad you are well."

"And looking forward to some wonderful cooking I am sure."

She smiled.

"You will be wanting to see him. Now?"

"Yes, I think so."

Climbing the main stairway, we walked down the second floor hallway to my father's office. The door was closed, but light showed under the door. I knocked twice then slowly opened the door. My father sat at his desk, head down, reading a book. An electric lamp on the desk providing a remarkable level of light.

"Father?"

He looked up from his book, took off his reading glasses and stood slowly.

"My God, David."

I extended my hand, but he took me in a bear hug. A solid grip told me that not only was he happy to see me, he was still the powerful man I had known all my life. It gave me a warm feeling of security, that a man of my age and experience should not need.

"You look well," I said, a little awkward.

"And you are a sight for sore eyes," he said, either ignoring or not seeing the scars on my face.

"This call for a drink," he said, walking to the credenza that served as a small bar. "Have you had anything to eat?"

"Not yet," I said.

Almost as if choreographed, Mrs. Randolph knocked then opened the door with a tray of sandwiches.

One toast, one sandwich and the two of us sat back, the only sound the light crackle of the fire in his small fireplace.

"So, tell me what's going on, are you on leave."

"I am, three weeks."

"But I read of the great Somme offensive, you weren't you part of that?"

I thought for a moment. How do I describe what had happened?

"The battalion took part in the first five days of the battle. Father, we lost almost five hundred dead, wounded and missing," I said. As an old soldier, he would understand.

"Five hundred? My God, how can that be? In five days?"

"I think war has changed from when you saw it. The machine guns and artillery wipe out the infantry as they try to advance. Rumors I heard before I left mentioned sixty thousand casualties on the first day."

"There's been nothing like that reported it the press."

"Father, I was there, I saw it."

He sat back in his high backed chair, his eyes unfocused on anything in the room. I am sure he was trying to connect what he knew of war with what I had said.

After a minute, he came back to the moment and said, "Tell me about your work in the field."

For two hours I described in detail the things I had seen in two years that I knew he would want to know as a physician. His questions told me he had been keeping up with the evolving techniques and science. We both finally said good night at midnight, spent from hours reliving my last two years.

The next morning, I awoke in a different world. For the last two years, rising had meant immediate tasks, either for maintenance of myself or taking care of patients. Now, I rested in a comfortable bed, surrounded by quiet, knowing I would be taken care of by the house staff. My solace lasted about ten minutes until I was compelled to get out of bed and begin my day, although I had no idea what that day might bring.

Mrs. Randolph outdid herself at breakfast, having Ellie, our cook, serve smoked kippers, soft-boiled eggs, venison sausage and oatcakes. It was a delight, but I found my ability to tuck in to a large breakfast seemed to have waned while in France. But the coffee was superb. A Jamaican Blue Mountain, it made the coffee in France pale in comparison. I would be taking some back with me when time came.

My father was just finishing his morning routine and leaving for the clinic when I came down. His invitation to visit the clinic was graciously declined as I had a mission to satisfy my own curiosity. But I did ask him if I might use the Daimler to take me about the town.

Long a fan of the automobile, my father purchased a Daimler in 1912 and directed our houseman, Richard Jordan, to learn to drive. The ability to get to patients without dealing with horses made his life much easier and truth be known, he loved the speed. I could drive well enough, but I thought there was no reason to test my ability when Richard knew exactly what he was doing on the road.

Maryhill Barracks served as the home depot for the Highland Light Infantry. Built in the 1870's, there was also a contingent of cavalry and artillery generally assigned as well. I had been to the barracks when my commission arrived, but spent little time there. The operations were overseen by Lieutenant Colonel Richardson, who at 60 years of age, was now relegated to watching the home fires as it were. New recruits were trained there, supplies coordinated and support for wounded soldiers provided. I wanted to see what was happening for my own edification.

Only a thirty minute drive from the house, it was interesting for me to see the activity on the streets as the people of Glasgow went about their daily rounds. Arriving at the Maryhill gate, a private saw my uniform and saluted.

"Sir?"

"I'm Captain McFadden, here to see Colonel Richardson."

"Yes, sir. His office is on the second floor of the main building."

There was a reasonable level of activity as I walked toward Richardson's office. Not really sure what I should be seeing, I could only compare it with the daily operations of the battalion. Individual soldiers walking down the corridors and soldiers at desks in offices all appeared to be hard at work. But I did wonder what their tasks must include.

I found the colonel's office, the outer area manned by an elderly sergeant smoking a pipe and reading a newspaper.

"Hello, I'm Captain McFadden of the second battalion, here to see the colonel."

The sergeant rose, putting his pipe in the tray and closing the paper.

"McFadden, you say, sir. Was the colonel expecting you?"

"No, I don't have an appointment. I just arrived from France and wanted to pay my respects."

He smoothed his uniform and walked toward the inner door.

"Just a minute, sir."

From the other room I heard, "McFadden, really? France? Send him in."

Shown in, I saluted and removed my cap.

"David McFadden, medical officer for the second."

"Yes, of course, please sit down, doctor."

Richardson was in his sixties I guessed, but well turned out and quite military in his stature.

"Just back from France?"

"Yes, sir. I left the battalion four days ago."

"You were there for the offensive?"

"I was, yes, sir."

He looked at me, started to say something then caught himself.

"It was a very difficult time," I said.

"The numbers I have seen are… hard to comprehend," he said.

"The Germans were well dug in with artillery and machine guns. Infantry charges simply do not make sense in those conditions."

"How is Colonel Abernathy? He was one of my subalterns many years ago."

"He is doing his duty, sir. Thank God he was spared in the battle. It will take a man of his ability to rebuild the battalion."

Richardson nodded.

"We have been told that our replacements will come from across the country. Gone are the days of local units I'm afraid."

What will that be like, I wondered. Men from all over England ordered into a Scottish regiment. The war had become too large and the need to man the army too voracious. How long do wars continue, until there are no more men to call up?

We talked about some of the issues I thought he could address and he dutifully took notes. It was time to leave and I asked him if there was any message I could carry back to the battalion.

He thought for a moment then said, "Make sure young Abernathy knows that we will do anything here to support him that we can. He must know that."

"I will, sir."

"When will you go back?"

"I have three weeks. Perhaps a week here in Glasgow and then I thought I would visit Queen Mary's Hospital in Roehampton. They are working with our men who have lost limbs and I want to see what they are doing."

"Ah, I see."

He stood up and offered his hand.

"Good luck, captain."

I saluted and took my leave.

My father was disappointed when I told him of my plans to visit Queen Mary's Hospital. But his medical instincts took over and he realized he would have done the same thing.

We were able to spend almost a week together and had opportunities to discuss the war, medicine and the future. I think those talks make my trip home worthwhile in themselves. I had not really thought about the future and his thoughts and advice were most welcome. Father and son became friends and comrades. Not a bad result for anyone in my estimation.

It struck me that I might go via Edinburgh on my way to London in the chance I could see Kathleen. I knew her address and the more I thought about her, the more I couldn't wait to get on the road. How would things between us be, away from the front and the war? I know I felt relaxed and the exhaustion that I thought had become permanent was actually gone. How would the time away affect her? I hoped her family was more accommodating than they had been when she left for France.

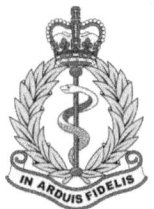

Chapter Twenty-Five

"You will always have a family."

England
3 July 1916

A short ride in a Hansom cab took me from Waverly Station to the North British Hotel on Prince Street. Recommended by my father, it was a remarkably luxurious hotel. I was able to book a suite with its own bathroom. Electric lights were the primary source of lighting after dark and there was even central heating, obviating the need for fireplaces which was fine with me. I was able to get a wonderful meal in the dining room and after a nightcap in the lounge I enjoyed a truly good night's sleep. It is interesting that two years ago, a sleep was not high on my list of desirables. Now there were few things I valued more. Perhaps I was entering the later stage of life early due to the war. I guess stranger things were possible.

I engaged a driver for the trip to Roslin, which I estimated at fifteen miles. The summer weather was enjoyable, but I found myself nervous as we approached the small town.

Kathleen told me a few things about her home and it appeared to be the ideal small Scottish town. Roslin was far enough away from the big city that it maintained a village like appearance. Having grown up in Glasgow proper, I appreciated the quiet and orderliness of the small villages that dotted the Scottish landscape.

Her address was listed as "Newcastle Lane," with no further description. In these small towns, everyone knew everyone else, including the postman, so no street numbers were needed.

My driver found Newcastle Lane after stopping to ask directions. A small sign identified the turn off the main road that led into a small valley. The first house we saw was just off the road, with a large orchard behind the house. There was a man in the front yard working on a farm wagon.

We pulled in and I got out, waving at the man, who walked away from the wagon, wiping his hands on a rag.

"Good morning," I said.

"Aye, and to ya."

"I'm looking for the Summers house."

"Summers?"

"Yes, I'm going to see his daughter, Kathleen."

The man, gray hair and stooped back, looked back at me, shrugging his shoulders.

"You'll not find her there," he said.

"Why do you say that?

"She came home from the war, she's a nurse, ya know, and her da threw her out of the house."

"He what?"

The old man nodded.

"Don't know why, but that's what people are saying."

Thrown out of her house by her father, that was absurd. But I remembered what she said about her family's attitude toward her going to France.

We found the Summers' house about a mile down the road. A large two story house, there was no evidence of farming other activity like the other house on the lane had shown. Her family must be prosperous, which would make sense with her academic accomplishments.

When we stopped, I decided to leave my cap in the car. The uniform in itself will make it clear that I am part of the war effort and I wasn't sure what response that would bring.

A middle-aged woman in a green dress opened the door wide and stood with her hands clasped together.

"May I help you?"

"I am Captain David McFadden of the Royal Army Medical Corps. I am looking for Miss Kathleen Summers."

A tall man in a white shirt and tie walked up behind the woman.

"I am Judge Summers. She's not here. Nor do I expect her in the foreseeable future. May I ask what is you reason to seeking her out?"

"I worked with her in France and wanted to see how she was on her leave from the front."

His voice was strong, perhaps from the courtroom.

"She will not be returning to France and is confirming that with the BRC in London. Is there anything else?"

I looked at the woman whom I suspected to be her mother. Her gaze was past me as if she was trying to distance herself from the words of her husband.

Judge Summers' face was a blank, showing no emotion one way or another. For a moment I entertained speaking my mind, but quickly realized it would be a waste of effort and likely to make things worse for Kathleen."

"No, sir. I think not. I am sorry for interrupting your day."

As I walked back to the car, a middle-aged man walked around the corner of the house. He was pushing a barrow and the implements therein told me he was likely a gardener. I stopped as he moved down the gravel pathway which paralleled the driveway.

"Excuse me."

He smiled at me.

"Military man, we don't see many around here."

"I was looking for Miss Kathleen Summers."

"Not here, I'm afraid. Left for London three days ago. I drove her to the station."

The morning express to London left Waverly Station at 7:00 sharp. Stopping at Charing Cross Station, it was near both my intended hotel and the headquarters of the British Red Cross on Pall Mall. It seemed like the best place to start my search. I am sure that if Kathleen was going to London, she would at least check in with the BRC, even if her ultimate destination was somewhere else in the city. I would find her, one way or the other. I still had almost two weeks of leave, and nothing was more important now that I learned of what her family had done.

"Oh yes, doctor. She's staying at the Cavendish Hotel on Jermyn street."

The full uniform, with cap served to solicit a most welcoming attitude from the receptionist. When I mentioned that we had worked together in France and had some official follow up business from the Royal Army Medical Corps, she could not have been more cooperative.

"Thank you, Miss. I shall try to catch her there. If I miss her, would you tell her Doctor McFadden has the papers she must sign following her time at the front in France. I am staying at the Savoy."

"She was at the front?" came with a rather surprised look.

"Yes, miss. The Battle of the Somme. She is quite a brave lady."

As I walked the short distance to Jermyn street, I thought about what I had said. She was certainly a very brave woman."

"Sir, her key is missing, so my assumption is that she is out."

The Cavendish was a modest hotel to say the least. Surprising to have a relatively low rent hotel in what could be described as one of the more upscale neighborhoods of London. Perhaps the BRC had some assignments for members staying in the capital and visiting the headquarters.

"Might I leave her a note?"

The man pushed a single piece of paper and an inkwell to me.

KATHLEEN,
I AM IN LONDON. I MUST SEE YOU. I WILL RETURN THIS EVENING, HOPING YOU HAVE RETURNED. IF WE MISS EACH OTHER, I AM AT THE SAVOY, ROOM 404.
LOVE, DAVID

A borne settee on one side of the lobby looked like a pleasant place to consider my next move and I walked over, taking a seat. My watch told me it was just before 6:00 pm and perhaps a drink was in order. As I looked around for a bar, there she was walking in the main entrance. It was the first time I had seen her in civilian clothes, and it took my breath away.

I walked across the lobby, and she didn't see me from the side as she approached the front desk.

"Kathleen."

She turned to me, hesitated for just a moment and then smiled. Her eyes twinkled and she held her arms out.

Public display of affection be damned, I took her in my arms.

"Oh, David."

We held each other for a moment then parted.

Looking down, I kissed her lightly on the lips and led her over to the settee.

"Tell me what happened?"

Sitting up very straight, she bowed her head then looked at me.

"David, I didn't understand how angry they were at my decision to go to France. My father is a very hard and strict man and to have his daughter defy him like that…I guess was too much."

Her hands were clasped in her lap as if she was getting ready to testify in court.

"I was told that my service with the Red Cross was at an end. Returning to Roslin and resuming a normal life was the only course open to me."

"I saw your father at the front door. He said you were not returning to France, but nothing about giving up nursing."

"That was understood. Live by their rules or I would not be part of the family."

What a bastard, I thought. To dictate to your daughter to live the life they planned or be disowned was unthinkable in this day and age.

I took her hands in mine.

"You will always have a family," I said.

She looked at me with a question in her eyes.

"I know our friendship is something I can always count on," she said and smiled.

My thoughts went to the discussion my father and I had about the future. Then I remembered holding her that night after the Somme, in that darkest of nights for England. I think my mind was already made.

"I don't mean our friendship, dearest."

There was a question in her eyes, perhaps some confusion, so I took the step.

"Kathleen, will you be my wife?"

"David, I."

"Miss Summers, I think I loved you from the moment I saw you in Rouen. The time we spent together only made me more convinced there is no woman I would rather spend the rest of my life with."

"And I do love you," she said after a moment. "I truly do, with all my heart. This thing with my family has me in such a birl."

"I would be confused as well. But it's your life and your future, not theirs."

Kathleen took both of my hands.

"Then, yes, my dear David. I will be your wife, and I will love you til the end of days."

Telegram to Doctor Lennox McFadden, Glasgow:

"Arriving evening train tomorrow with fiancé, Kathleen Summers. Please arrange small wedding ceremony, St. Andrew's Cathedral, Friday, 7th, time your discretion. Plan brief honeymoon to Barr Loch over weekend, then returning London. David."

That evening we enjoyed dinner in the Savoy Grill. While I tried to have Kathleen move to the Savoy, she said that for only one night it made no sense. I think she felt in unfamiliar territory as we were shown to our table, but she was smiling and had taken my arm. I was a most happy man.

I knew my father would support my decision, despite the multitude of issues many would say make my decision crazy. There was the war, certainly, but I was most aware of the dangers of life at the front. Our religious differences might be another issue, but I didn't see it. I'd already decided to convert if Kathleen desired it. The Church of England, regardless of history, was closer to Catholicism than most. Besides, I knew of a larger than life Catholic priest who would happily provide me instruction. The reaction of her family would surely be an issue for now and years to come, but there was nothing I could do about it and so I wasn't going to worry.

"This is lovely," she said looking around the room.

"It is always a pleasure to visit the grill when in London."

"Isn't it frightfully expensive?"

"I guess it is, but the food and service are certainly worth it and I think this is a very special occasion. In fact, I do believe a bottle of champagne would suit well."

She looked a bit surprised.

"I've never had champagne."

"Really, then what spirit do you find the most agreeable?"

"Oloroso sherry in public, Campbeltown Scotch in private."

"One more reason why I love you, Kathleen Summers."

A bottle of Louis Roederer, 1904, could not have been a better accompaniment to the dinner.

We both chose fillet of sole, after so much beef at the front. A delightful dinner finished with a remarkable peach melba.

Over coffee, we made small talk about nothing, just enjoying talking to each other. Too many conversations in the last year had dealt with life and death, now was the time to revel in happiness.

"It seems you are accustomed to quite a luxurious life style."

I didn't comment as our second cups of coffee were being poured. The waiter nodded and moved off.

"The new doctor, just starting out, just making ends meet?'

"Something like that," she said.

"My father has a well-established practice in Glasgow, which I hope to take over some day. But no, it wasn't medicine. My grandfather started the largest private bank in Glasgow in 1855. We still own the majority share."

"But you went into medicine, not banking."

"Never any question. I think watching my father and how he helped people grabbed my imagination at a very young age."

Kathleen smiled. "I read a book about Florence Nightingale when I was a young girl. From then on, I wanted to be a nurse. Funny how those things happen."

I thought of Kathleen ministering to wounded soldiers at the front. Florence would be proud.

"I'm glad it did, Nurse Summers."

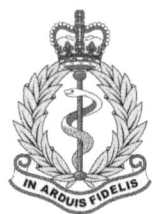

Chapter Twenty-Six

"It is my husband, now I am happy."

Glasgow
July 1916

My father and Mrs. Randolph were standing on the platform when our train slowly came to a stop in Glasgow. Steam and the smell of oil permeated the air, and the passengers moved en masse toward the lobby. I waited just a moment for the crowd to clear and we stepped on the platform. My father raised his hat, although I was already walking to where they stood with Kathleen on my arm.

As we approached, he removed his hat and extended his hand to Kathleen.

"Father, Miss Kathleen Summers," I said formally.

He smiled broadly.

"Kathleen, I'm Lennox McFadden. A most warm welcomed to Glasgow."

Kathleen took his hand and returned his smile.

"Doctor McFadden, it is my pleasure to finally meet you."

I intervened.

"Dear, this is Mrs. Julia Randolph."

"Mrs. Randolph, David has told me so much about you."

"Kathleen, while David insists on calling me Mrs. you must call me Julia. Welcome, welcome."

"Richard is waiting for us," my father said.

I hailed a porter and with our bags in tow, our happy group left the station.

The ride to the house was dedicated to a tour of Glasgow. My father took the lead, with a steady description of the sights. I was surprised at his knowledge of the city and Kathleen could not have been more attentive. Father was clearly enjoying himself.

On arrival, after a quick freshen up, we gathered in the parlor.

"Why do you insist on calling Julia, Mrs. Randolph?" Kathleen asked once we were all settled.

"Well, when I was twelve, my father told me that as far as he was concerned, I was a man. As such, I would decide what clothes to wear, when to go to bed, what I would eat, pretty much everything. But his guidance was that to maintain his trust I must show common sense, humility and frugality. Quite a challenge for a twelve year old. One of the things I decided was that anyone older than me would be addressed formally. I have continued that to this day."

"Oh, my," Kathleen said, "That is wonderful."

"And I can't wait to call you Mrs. McFadden," I said winking at her.

Father said, "Speaking of that, would you like to go over the arrangements now or wait until after dinner?"

Kathleen looked at me and I got the message.

"I think we both would like to go over them now," I said.

"Very well. Archbishop Mackintosh will preside over the ceremony. He's been a patient for many years and he was very helpful with this rather impromptu wedding. Mixed marriages are not encouraged by the Catholic Church, but as long as the non-Catholic agrees to allow the spouse to worship as a Catholic and raise any children in the church, they are permitted. The only rule that he could not change was that the ceremony must take place in the rectory, not the main chapel."

"That is not a problem," I said, relieved that there wasn't something that was going to prohibit our marriage.

"With the ceremony so soon, have you thought about who might be invited and what you will wear?"

"Doctor McFadden, David and I have discussed this."

My father held up his hand.

"My dear, you are about to become part of this family. Please call me Lennox, or if you are so inclined I would be grateful if you were to call me father."

Kathleen rose and walked over to him. She bent down and kissed his forehead.

"Thank you, father."

I felt a warmth and calm like never before. How could I be so lucky.

I spoke up.

"Father, we would like the ceremony to be just our household. During this time of war, privacy is important to us. And we decided that I will wear my uniform as will Kathleen."

"A splendid plan, splendid."

"O God, who by your mighty power created all things out of nothing, and when you had set in place the beginnings of the universe, formed man and woman in your own image, making the woman an inseparable helpmate to the man... Pour out the grace of the Holy Spirit on this your daughter Kathleen, and on this your servant David, that, as they begin their married life, they may be strengthened by your blessing."

Donald Mackintosh was gracious and welcoming. The ceremony was a very comfortable thirty minutes. His words and the gospel he chose matched perfectly.

Kathleen could not have been lovelier, having taken a bit of freedom to have her hair down instead of up in a bun which was the normal Red Cross standard. While her hair did slightly cover her scars, I know now that she had no shame or concern that she would ever show the wounds of the war. One more reason why I loved her so much.

While this was a very happy occasion, she had been quiet and attentive during the time leading up to the ceremony. I wondered if it was because she was thinking about her family. Someday we would come to grips with that situation, but now we had our lives to get on with.

Rather than a reception, which made no sense, we invited the archbishop to lunch at the Willow Tea Room. It was exactly what was called for, a perfect lunch of roast pheasant with bread sauce and game chips. As I enjoyed the meal, I thought of the cans of bully beef that waited for me in France. Ah, well. Enjoy it while you can.

That afternoon Mr. Jordan had the car ready, and we waved goodbye to father and Mrs. Randolph.

I took Kathleen's hand, and we sat in the back seat watching the scenery, but not saying anything. There was a comfort I felt and I'm sure she did also. The ceremony went quite well and the lunch was warm and friendly. Perhaps she would start to heal from the wound by her family.

The afternoon sun had begun to fade as we turned off the main road, heading west toward Barr Loch. My family had maintained a fishing lodge here for as long as I could remember. Father was an avid angler and I'll admit I found myself enjoying it more as I got older.

Thirty minutes on a winding road brought us to the waterfront, dock and lodge. A one-story wooden house, it had a large rock chimney at the northern end. A wide veranda faced the loch and a large gazebo stood in the side lawn.

Kathleen and I had declined to have any assistance from the staff, wanting to finally have time together. Mr. Jordan opened the lodge and brought in our bags and several boxes of supplies which Mrs. Randolph had put together. An ice chest was also part of our supply train, and included delicacies and two bottles of champagne. His final duty was to light the candles around the lodge.

The sun would be down in about an hour and my thought was to have a drink and watch the sunset. As it turned out, events took over and we missed the sunset entirely.

When I opened my eyes, the sun was already painting a shadow on the wall. Kathleen was not there, her side of the bed neatly arranged as I would have expected.

I found her in the main room in one of the high back wing chairs that faced the loch. She was wrapped in a shawl, her nightdress covering her feet. Turning her head, I watched her eyes soften and a wispy smile appear.

"It is my husband, now I am happy."

She reached for me, and we closed our arms around each other.

We kissed and Kathleen asked with a twinkle in her eyes, "Do you always sleep so late?"

"Dreams of last night kept me blissfully asleep. But now that I am up and about, I should think about putting together a hearty breakfast."

"Perhaps oat cakes and tea?"

"Not much of a challenge to my culinary prowess, but yes, oak cakes and tea it shall be, with Mrs. Randolph's raspberry preserves."

After the events of our time in England, it was a wonderful luxury to have nothing of need to accomplish. Our time was filled with talking, walking, one sortie on the loch and a nature walk. But the calendar was very clear, both of us were due to return to France in the next week. For the first day, we were two young newly weds and acted as such. After the last two years, I found it totally delightful and knew our decision to marry was the right one, regardless of what the future held. I'd talked with so many soldiers who put marriage on hold because of the war. It made sense to me at the time. But now I could not agree. If there is love, marriage is simply the declaration. Nothing in the future should detract from that. Perhaps a too simplistic view, but it was sensible to this humble soldier.

The last evening, we were watching the late afternoon sun move across the loch and having a drink. I decided to broach a subject I had given a great deal of thought and now was ready to raise with Kathleen.

"I would like for you to consider a change when you return to France."

She looked surprised.

"A change?"

"You spent a very long time on the front lines with the battalion."

"I did. Where is this going?" she asked.

I knew I must be circumspect, but still make my point.

"You've seen German artillery, and I don't want you in harm's way again."

"What are you saying?"

"I'm asking you to take a position in a field hospital, away from the front."

Kathleen was quiet for a long minute.

"Away from your surgical team?"

"Yes. Not that I don't want you by my side, but the chance you might be wounded or killed would be too much for me. I don't think I could do my job as I know I have to."

"Then come with me to a field hospital. Your surgical skills would be welcome at any of them. It would give you a chance to do more surgery in a year than most in a lifetime. You certainly know the value of that."

She was right, by every measure. And my argument was weak on the surface, but powerful to me.

"You're right and I know you are. But I want this surgical team idea to work and to do that I have to keep it going. Also, there's the battalion. I've been with them for two years. They're part of me even if that makes no sense."

Looking out at the loch, she said, "Yes, my dear, unfortunately it makes all the sense in the world after being there with you."

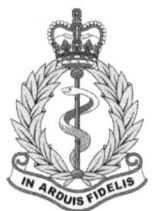

Chapter Twenty-Seven

"The Hun artillery only gets worse."

Le Havre
1 August 1916

My thoughts returned to my arrival in France almost two years ago. The harbour and quayside demonstrated the remarkable expansion of everything dealing with the war. More troops, truck, cargo and confusion. Walking down the gangway, I carried one small duffel and purposefully made my way to the RTO's office. For some reason I found myself getting angry, but didn't know why. Was the reality of returning to a world of pain and death taking hold? Or was it the parting with Kathleen after such a short time as man and wife. Perhaps I was just getting old.

"McFadden, left the Highland Light's three weeks ago. Have they moved?"

An officious major looked up from his desk, with an annoyed look. He was about to say something then saw the ribbon on my tunic.

"Highland Lights, let me check."

Looking around it struck me nothing had changed in two years. I found that discouraging.

"Here it is. They are at the Corbie Depot. That is just east of Amiens."

"Best way to get there?" I asked.

"You're in luck. I have a troop train leaving here in an hour. It'll take you to Amiens. Transport from there should be no problem."

"Do I need authorization?"

"I'll fill it out right now."

He pulled a sheet of paper from one of many piles and began to write.

"Damn, I forgot. There's no officer's coach on that train, just boxcars for the troops."

"I don't care, riding with the lads is fine."

He looked askance at me, but the hell with him. I took my authorization and headed for the railhead.

I well knew of the famous French "40 et 8" boxcars, designed for 40 men or 8 horses, riding in very close quarters. But I wanted to get back to the battalion and comfort be damned.

Finding the railhead was not the problem. But multiple tracks contained different trains, all seemingly ready to pull out. The noise of coupling mechanisms, steam release and whistles attested to the controlled chaos that seemed to always pervade any crossroads. Seeing a British sergeant with an armband and signaling flag I was able to get to my train, which was identified by "XR32" scrawled in chalk on each of eight boxcars. I walked down the tracks looking in the doors and found the third car seemed to have the most room.

I laid my duffel on the car floor and asked the men by the door to help me up. Several hands pulled me aboard, the men steadying me as the train was bumped by an engine or another car.

"My name's McFadden. Hitching a ride to Amiens with you lads if you're good with that."

Several men looked surprised. I assume they weren't used to having a captain ask permission of them for anything. I found a spot for my bag and sat down on what looked like fresh straw.

The men on each side were clearly new recruits on their way to the front for the first time. My God, what they must be thinking. How many of them would never see England again?

A double whistle and the jerk from the engine began our journey. The clear sky and warm weather promised a pleasant trip, assuming the German's did not find the train with their aircraft. I could only hope that our own Royal Flying Corps was up and about today.

During the five hour journey to Amiens I discovered that the men in my car were all going to the Lancashire Fusiliers. I recalled that their first and second battalions had been particularly hard hit on the first day of the attack. The men had been training at the infantry base depot outside of Le Havre. The war's insatiable need for more manpower had begun to overwhelm the normal training route used by the army for many years. It made me wonder if the men I saw training in Glasgow would make it to the battalion or be swept off to where the need was the greatest. This war continues to change the world we had all known, and likely not for the good.

A lucky encounter with an ambulance caravan provided a ride back to the battalion, now in reserve near the town of Contay. Talking with my ambulance driver, it was clear the bloody offense was continuing. I suddenly felt uneasy. Had the battalion gone back into action without their medical officer?

I knew our battalion needed literally hundreds of replacements, but if the situation was critical, would the high command send a skeleton battalion back into the trenches?

The rest area near Contay was large. As we approached in our ambulance, I saw many rows of tents, certainly more than a battalion. The driver thought there were several battalions in the area, but didn't know for sure. I thanked him and walked to the nearest row of tents with my duffel.

"Looking for the Highland Lights," I said, on seeing two sergeants outside of a large tent.

"Far west side of the camp, captain."

In fifteen minutes, I began to see familiar faces and then the regimental colors at the end of a row of tents. I was home as it were.

"The prodigal son has returned," James said as I stuck my head into the tent.

He was on his cot, a magazine open on his chest.

"Certainly where I would expect to find an Englishman," I laughed and we shook hands.

"You look well, David, the time away did you good."

"So well in fact that I was married ten days ago."

James sat up, a surprised look on his face.

"Kathleen and I, in Glasgow."

"Good lord, that I did not expect."

I explained the events that led up to our marriage and how I was happier than I could have ever imagined.

"Where's she now?" he asked.

"Posted to the field hospital at Boulogne. She wasn't happy to leave the battalion or the surgical team, but she did it for me."

"That is good, my friend. The Hun artillery only gets worse. She would be in danger up here."

I started unpacking my duffel and James updated me on the battalion. We have received about two hundred replacement troops. The issue was replacing our junior officers, the platoon commanders. We lost nine during our week on the line with only two new lieutenants reporting to replace them. While we lost sergeants, an experienced corporal was expected to move up in the ranks. I didn't recall seeing any lieutenants at Maryhill Barracks during my time in Glasgow. Perhaps we would get our replacement officers from other regiments.

"We are going to lose Abernathy," James said. "He is being promoted to full colonel and moved up to the Fifth Brigade staff."

"Who is going to replace him?" I asked, sorry to hear he was leaving. While I had little experience with battalion commanders, it is hard to imagine a better man and soldier than Colonel Abernathy."

"Apparently, his name in Prescott, Abner Prescott. He's the senior major in the First Battalion and is being promoted to Lieutenant Colonel and moved to Second Battalion."

"Heard anything about him?"

"Sergeant Nance told me Prescott is known to be a stickler for rules and regulations."

"We shall just have to take things as they come."

In fact, the arrival of Lieutenant Colonel Abner Prescott was similar to a German artillery barrage. On the day of his arrival, there were two staff meetings, one full battalion parade and companywide equipment inspections.

My one on one interview did not take place until the second day. But it only added to my opinion that our new battalion commander was convinced that he knew more about any and everything than anyone else in the command.

After being told that half of my efforts must be directed toward the cleanliness of the men, food and shelter, Prescott proceeded to lecture me on the problems with casualty evacuation procedures. He expected an expeditious and orderly movement of any wounded to the nearest casualty clearing station. He did not think the concept of a battalion aid station made any sense as the purpose of front line medical personnel was to get the wounded away from the front as quickly as possible.

Rather than explain our surgical team capability, I simply nodded my acknowledgment of his direction and left after a frustrating twenty minutes.

If I was a new doctor, I might have bought into what Prescott was saying. But I had two years of front line experience and he had spent most of the last two years on the brigade staff that oversaw the First Battalion.

I would continue to do my job, take care of our troopers and stay away from Abner Prescott.

That afternoon, I met with all of the medical staff. It was good to see them all together. We had luckily avoided any serious injuries to our doctors or medical orderlies. Thank goodness our senior stretcher bearer, Jimmy Chesney had survived so far unharmed. Not so with the other bearers, we had lost seven of our core group.

I made it clear that we were going to continue doing business just as we have in the past. I wanted Jimmy, Corey and Jonesy to conduct a crash course for our new bearers. I expected we would be moving back into the line within the next ten days. The offensive had become fragmented with specific areas under attack in a continuing attempt to force a break in the German lines. Thank God, the front wide attack was a thing of the past, at least for now.

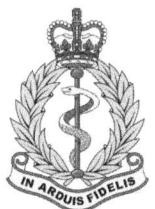

Chapter Twenty-Eight

"Doc, we need you."

Southwest of Courcelette
14 September 1916

While still one hundred soldiers understrength, the Second Battalion had been ordered to move up in preparation for a coordinated attack on the town of Courcelette. The attacking force would include, British, French and Canadians. In another step forward in warfare, a new invention, an armoured tractor, would take part in the attack. Developed by our army, the steel monsters were called "tanks," by headquarters and it was hoped they would sweep barbed wire and machine gun positions aside as they moved across the battlefield. In the typical give and take of warfare, we had also been told the Germans were introducing a new aircraft that was said to be superior to anything we or the French are currently flying. The insanity continues.

The companies were all working with new command structures and we were still short platoon commanders. I was lucky to have our old medical staff with the exception of Kathleen and Alice Bradbury. The Red Cross pulled Alice back to the military hospital at Rouen because of a severe shortage of nurses. The move meant that Jonesy would become my main surgical assistant. Quite a journey by the former dispatch rider turned medical orderly.

Jonesy had been rather subdued since we both returned from leave. I tried to sound out his change in demeanor, but he seemed reticent to discuss. I had to respect our long time together and let it go. He will be a superb surgical assistant, having worked very well with Glen Rossi through many procedures.

The Canadian doctor was a superb member of the team. Consistently positive, he took any challenge in stride, no matter how difficult. Perhaps it was the Canadian frontier spirit, quite different from the traditional English approach to almost everything.

As the sun was going down, James, Rand and I walked down to the main trench area with Corporals Timmons and Ennis. We were able to find two good positions for the aid stations, relatively protected by the rolling terrain. Timmons and Ennis would bring down the bearers and erect tarp covers and fill sandbags to provide shelter in the event of artillery fire.

All I needed now was to set up our surgical tent and make sure we were ready for business.

Having been away from the front for three weeks, the artillery barrage took me by surprise. It seemed that the number of guns continued to grow every time there was a barrage. I did notice the stockpile of shells during our move to the new location and it was difficult to take in. There must have been thousands of shells of all calibers. The time, effort and cost to build up those supplies must have been astronomical. And all they would accomplish was to kill men and destroy the land. It seemed more ludicrous whenever I thought about it. But I wasn't going to change anything, I just have to take care of the battalion. Focus on our job and don't worry about the bigger picture.

Twenty minutes after our barrage began in the predawn, we begin to get return fire from the Germans. While the impacts seemed to concentrate on the front lines, numerous explosions erupted up and down the lines. It brought home to me why I didn't want Kathleen anywhere near the front.

The attack was scheduled to begin at 0730, with the troops following a creeping barrage. In the last two years, our artillery had developed the ability to move the impacts across no man's land in front of our troops.

The hope was to destroy the enemy trenches, but also to keep the Germans under cover as our lads advanced.

The bivouac was almost deserted except for our medical tent and some of the cooks. Several ambulances were standing by and ready to transport any wounded to the CCS. Being only several hundred yards from the main line, the attack was evident at 0730 as the sounds of automatic fire began to echo across the fields. The ongoing artillery fire contributed to a non-stop cacophony of destruction. I knew the results of that clash would start to arrive in short order.

Our first seven casualties were wounded by artillery shells before they left the trenches. While the use of the new Brodie helmet had cut down on some shrapnel injuries, the metal would not provide protection from rifle or machine gun bullets unless the strike was a glancing blow. But any protection was better than none and even the medical staff had been issued their own helmets.

Side impacts from exploding shells were uniformly dangerous and often lethal. Some of the shell fragments were several inches across, large enough to do major damage to a limb or torso. The small fragments, while not often fatal could be totally incapacitating due to the loss of blood and shock of impact.

Our first casualties did not require any additional care other than more or better bandages and saline solution. We were able to get them on the ambulances and on their way to the CCS in very little time. I have come to the conclusion that rapid care is the key to survival in this brand of medicine. Minimal surgery unless the patient's survival dictates intervention. The trauma of transportation is also of key importance. A motor ambulance is often key due to the speed of transport, although the speed often increases the roughness of the ride which can make a difference. A slow and steady horse driven ambulance, while much more stable it can take five times as long to get the patient to the CCS. If we have options, we will direct the patient go by motor ambulance if the loss of blood or respiratory problems are pronounced. Each patient must be evaluated for all aspects of his treatment if we are doing our job correctly.

As we cleaned up from our first casualties, Jimmy Chesney rushed into the medical prep area. He looked across at me, his face covered by sweat, his face reflecting shock.

"Jimmy.."

"The aid station's gone, it's gone, they're all dead!"

I looked at him, then what he said began to hit me. I walked across the tent and grabbed him by both arms.

"Jimmy, what do you mean?"

"A direct hit, there's nothing left, no people, nothing. The doc, everyone just gone."

"Who," I yelled at him.

"Doc Edwards, Ennis, Tisdale's whole team, they're gone."

I realized what Jimmy had said, but my mind tried to reject it. He was upset and needed to calm down, that was something I could do.

"Jimmy, sit down. Ryan, get him a cigarette."

Christ.

Do your job. Now more than ever.

"Jimmy, you're telling me that the aid station is no longer there?

He nodded.

"My God," was all I could say. But I needed to deal with what had happened. The attack was underway, and they needed medical support.

"Glen, you stay here with Dan. Do what you can and keep the wounded going to the CCS. I'm going down to set up another aid station. Ryan, get some medical bags together, we leave as soon as we can."

My helmet and pistol were with my tunic in the back. That's all I would need, that and plenty of morphine. Christ, James was dead.

We jogged toward the trench lines, artillery shells exploding along the front. I heard our artillery firing at the same time, the explosions and shrieks adding to the tumult. We reached where the aid station had been, a large crater was still smoking. Pieces of bandage, uniforms and body parts covered the ground, the smell of cordite strong and biting.

"Down there," I yelled, pointing to a small hill fifty yards west of us.

Jonesy picked up his bags and ran toward the hill, followed by Jimmy Chesney and his team, who were carrying two stretchers and more equipment.

Several small trees added to the cover behind the hill and we began to set up the aid station.

"Jimmy, get down and tell anyone you see where the new aid station is, then go get the boys who need us."

He nodded and his team moved off toward the sound of the machine guns.

"He was a good man," Jonesy said as we sat in the grass listening to the sounds of the attack.

What do you say when a friend dies? In battle it is expected, but he was a doctor. He was there to take care of wounded men. But I was not a fool. Doctors die just like chaplains and stretcher bearers.

"Yes, he was," I said. I thought about his wife and young son. The terrible news that would shatter their life. Like it had been happening to English families for two damned years. When was this terrible folly going to end, and what the hell was it accomplishing?

I saw Jimmy coming down the small valley from the trenches with two of his team right behind him.

"Doc, we need you," he yelled.

"What?"

"A dozen wounded. Jerry has them pinned down. They're in a big damn crater, but they need help. We can't get 'em out with the machine gun right on top of us."

I saw the look in his eyes. Jimmy was a veteran, but I could see he was upset.

"Right," I said, knowing what had to be done. I remembered my time in no man's land and pictured the wounded men. There was only one choice.

I pointed to two of our medical bags.

"Jimmy bring those along."

Jonesy was reaching for the bags.

"Ryan, I need you to stay here. Take care of the wounded and get them back to Rossi."

"But, doc."

"I need you here. Understand?"

He nodded.

"Let's go."

Jimmy led our small group down the ravine toward the entry to the trench system. The sounds of machine gun fire were constant, and I could tell from the sounds, it was Germans doing the firing.

We slipped into the reserve trench, which was 20 yards back from the primary trench. A communication trench ran forward, and we moved toward the opening. I stepped over a soldier lying on his back, a terrible bullet wound in his face. There were two other men in the trench, both had bandages evident.

"There's an aid station, a hundred yards up the ravine. Get up there and have the orderly look at you," I said as I walked by them.

"Doctor!"

As we approached the communication trench, I turned to see Lieutenant Colonel Prescott with a lieutenant aide and the sergeant major.

"Yes, sir."

"What is God's name are you doing down here?"

"We have wounded men pinned down out there, colonel."

"Send the bearers," he snapped.

"They're pinned down, sir. The bearers can't get them out right now and they need medical care."

"But you can't go out there," he said.

"Sir, I have to go, and I have to go right now."

I turned and motioned to Jimmy, who turned and headed down the comm trench.

"Doctor."

I heard the colonel, but ignored him.

"We'll go left of the big wire area. There's a path through the wire that's partially sheltered until we are about thirty yards from the lads. Stay as low as you can and if I hit the dirt, you do the same. Right?"

"Understood," I said, and I meant it.

He went on as we approached the ladder.

"I think there's one machine gun that's doing all the damage. Get ready and when a long burst ends, we go."

Jimmy climbed on the wooden ladder and I moved right behind him. His two bearers, who I recognized as Privates Austin and Woods were right behind be, each carrying a medical duffel. I had a haversack on my back, which kept both my hands free. For some odd reason that made me feel better. I could also feel my pistol in its holster on my right hip. While the RAMC did not condone the carrying of weapons, I didn't care. Just like I never wore my medical armband. I expected no consideration from the enemy, nor was I going to go foolishly into harm's way without protection.

Jimmy's third bearer was in charge of the stretcher. He had already slid it over the top of the trench to be able to grab it when it was time.

"Go…Go!" Jimmy called, pulling himself over the trench top. I got up the ladder as quickly as I could and started on hands and knees after Corporal Chesney.

As we moved forward, it was a bizarre combination of crawling, running in a crouch and sliding down into cover when the machine gun opened up. It seemed we were not being targeted and I could hear bullet impacts off to our left as we reached a relatively open area.

"Down," Jimmy called, and we all went to ground. The summer weather meant we were not dealing with mud, but the dust and smoke surely choked all of us.

My head was even with Jimmy's waist, and he turned to look at me.

"Thirty yards ahead. See the wooden post poking up to the right?"

I could see what looked like a rail tie sticking into the air.

"I see it."

"The lads are just on the other side of that. If we run toward the left side of that little hill, there's cover." Once you get there, roll over the top and you'll be in the crater."

"Right."

"You ready?" he asked.

I nodded, taking a deep breath.

For ten yards, nothing happened, and I stayed low, moving as fast as I could. Then the machine gun opened up, the bullets cracking past us, some ricochetting, others throwing up soil all around us.

There was nothing to do, but run and hope.

I made it to the crater, saw Jimmy roll over the edge and I went right after him. The machine gun stopped firing, maybe to reload, and both our privates followed us into the crater. Our stretcher carrier left the stretcher outside of the crater, rolling over the top with a cloud of dust.

We scrambled across the depression to the German facing side where the men were lying in the cover of the crater wall.

Several of the wounded men looked at us with surprise as the four of us tried to catch our breath. Thank the Lord, we had made it.

"Jimmy, how far are we from the German trench?"

He wiped his face with his sleeve.

"I make it a hundred yards, give or take."

I heard shots coming from our right.

"How many of our own men are out here?"

"A lot have gone to ground, some have retreated. Not sure how many, but there are pockets out here, just like us."

"Keep a watch, we don't need the Germans creeping up on us.

Now to take care of these men.

As quickly as I could, a cursory exam of each man told me where my priorities must lie.

Two of the men were dead, and one grievously wounded with multiple bullet wounds in his chest. The amount of blood was significant, and his ashen face told me that he had only a little time left. He was unconscious, his breathing thready. I had to let him go, there were eight other men of which five needed immediate attention.

"Jimmy, give me a hand here."

Kneeling next to a private with a compound fracture of his right thigh, I told Jimmy to find a board at least five feet long. I needed to stop the immediate bleeding, treat the pain and splint the leg in place to prevent more damage.

"What's your name?" I asked the man, whose head rested in his helmet, braced against the sloping side of the crater.

"Ainsley, Freddie Ainsley."

"I'll be working on your leg, but first put these two pills under your tongue for me."

The morphine would dull the pain of splinting and the tourniquet I was about to apply. Jimmy found a dirty board that likely came from a trench wall. Using several long bandages, I was able to put a steady pressure to keep the wound from opening up and doing more damage.

"Jimmy, wipe down his face when you can and give him a little water in about ten minutes,"

I moved past two men to a corporal who was already sporting several bloody bandages around his neck and head.

"Corporal, I'm Doctor McFadden. Let me take a look at your head."

As I gently moved the bandage I determined his last name was Brownely. The wound ran from his right eye back through the remains of the right ear. A furrow down to the white skull had bled profuse amounts of blood that ran down his neck into his tunic. Thank God it was just blood with no additional wounds. I had no Dakin's with me, but hoped the heavy bleeding had helped to cleanse the wound. I would note the wound needed thorough cleaning on his patient card. Two morphine tablets and a fresh bandage set him up well to wait for evacuation.

In the back of my mind, unless the German machine gun was destroyed, our only chance was to wait for the sun to go down and get these men out during darkness. With the sun still rising in the sky, we wouldn't see the sunset for at least another eight or nine hours. The sun would pay hell with the thirst of the men, particularly with their wounds.

Private Goode was next on my patient sheet, having half of his right hand shot away, leaving only the thumb and forefinger attached. I could see he was in severe pain and on the edge of panic.

"Private, I'm going to do everything I can right now, but the real work will have to be done in England."

Gritting his teeth, he tried to acknowledge what I said, but then closed his eyes and sobbed.

Again, morphine and bandages were in order, the pain level would increase as the day went on. We might not have much water, but morphine was not a problem. The wound was contaminated with dirt, indicating a level of water use that was hard to use, knowing our shortage. The shattered bone structure of the hand was very difficult to clean and would need to be done again at CCS, but I had to use some of our dwindling water supply.

Thankfully, the morphine was doing its work as I finished with the private and moved on.

My next two patients thankfully had simple bullet wounds, both in their lower legs. There was no bone damage or major vessel involvement. I hoped that both of them would be able to walk with assistance and not need to be carried on our way out of here. I asked Jimmy to try and rig up some type of cane for each of them.

That took care of the immediate needs, and I checked back to the first man I had examined. He had died while I was working on the others. That is a difficult thing to rationalize, and I hoped I would not have to deal with that choice again.

"Jimmy, we're going to need more water if we have to wait until dark."

"Right, doc."

"So, of your men, which one do you think can get out and back with replenished canteens?"

"Me."

I looked at the older corporal and knew he was right. But I hated the thought of not having him out here with me to deal with whatever might come up.

"Besides you."

He thought for a moment.

"Woody."

Ten minutes later, Private Woods scrambled over the far edge of the crater carrying six canteens. Either his move caught the Germans by surprise or they weren't going to waste ammunition on a single soldier. Now he can only make it back with the water.

Of my last three soldiers, two were very straightforward, a simple broken wrist and a severely sprained ankle. Appropriate immobilizing wraps took care of them with a small amount of morphine to dull the pain.

Finally, I moved over to my last charge. Private Sullivan had lain quietly while I treated all of his comrades. Having taken a quick look at him initially, it appeared to me that he had been the victim of a Minenwerfer, one of the small mortars the Germans used in the trenches. He had actually been lucky, the exploding shell had hit him with dirt and not shrapnel. Unfortunately the force of the explosion was into his face. Now he was unable to see. His comrades had bandaged his eyes and now I was going to see if there way anything I could do in the field to treat the damage.

Carefully I unwound the bandage covering his eyes. The remainder of his face was peppered with small wounds from dirt and rock fragments.

His eyes were closed and caked with the combination of drainage and dirt. I gently cleaned around the eyelids using water and gauze.

"Keep you eyes closed while I clean things up a bit."

"All right," he said quietly, grimacing at the pain.

"What's your first name private?"

"William, Bill."

"Well Bill, let's see what we've got here. Slowly open your eyes."

I watched the young man's face twitch and put my hand up to shade his eyes from the direct sun.

As his eyelids rose, the first impression was from the very red tone of the scelera, a sure sign of significant irritation. But then as I bent lower to examine his eyes, I could see both corneas were clear. In my experience, that foretold a positive outcome for for Private Sullivan. Only time would tell, but I would flush the eye and rebandage to keep the eyes under as little strain as possible.

With the obvious pain, I mixed cocaine powder to form an anesthetic solution. Dripping it into each eye provided quick relief for Private Sullivan. I was able to carefully clean each eye of the dirt and debris. While his eyes looked terrible, I felt we had avoided major damage. Having seen too many cases of blindness over the last two years, this was heartening to me.

"Ah, no major damage, but your eyes have taken a beating. I'll put the bandage back on and we'll get you to hospital. A good rest will do wonders."

I was not totally truthful, but for the here and now it served my purpose to get him back to our lines with the minimum of struggle.

Morphine was administered and in short order, Private Sullivan was resting comfortably as possible.

I moved over near Jimmy Chesney who was on his stomach, keeping watch on the area between our crater and the German trench.

"How are you doing, Jimmy."

"Quiet out there for now, doc. That machine gun is still in position, but they're just watching, it seems."

"You think they'd send patrols out?"

"Don't know. Maybe."

Reaching inside my tunic, I pulled out my watch. The bright gold flashed in the sun. My father gave it to me when I graduated from school. Manufactured by the J.W. Benson Company, it was a truly beautiful watch. I read the inscription as I opened it.

"Doctor David McFadden – 1910."

The dial told me that it was 1:22. I wish I had noted when Private Woods had left, but it seemed it had been about two hours. How long should it take I wondered, knowing how the challenges on the battlefield could alter the normal flow of everything.

Several of the men were using their helmets as a shade against the sun. Well, if it can't protect against rifle bullets, at least it can provide some cover from the sun. And the when time comes, I am sure it will be effective protection from the rain.

From up forward, the German machine gun opened fire after a prolonged quiet period. The fire was directed off to our right and I saw Woods returning, running in a crouch. Several other men were right behind him, running and staying as low as possible.

Then frustration of the day took over. I was angry. All we wanted was water for our wounded. I quickly stepped across the crater to where a Lee Enfield rifle lay next to Private Sullivan. I picked up the rifle and cycled the bolt, noting rounds in the magazine. Taking off my helmet, I eased up to the crater rim, sliding the rifle slowly over it. The rifle felt good in my hands and familiar. I had grown up hunting with my father and I knew how to use a rifle.

The German opened up again and I aimed just right of embrasure where I could see the distinctive barrel of the German MG 08. The barrel was surrounded by a light metal water jacket that kept the barrel from overheating. I could clearly see the front half of the water jacket and lined up my sights. Carefully squeezing the trigger, the rifle fired. I quickly worked the bolt, cycling another round into the chamber and aimed again at the jacket, noting the machine gun had ceased firing. Another round out of the Lee Enfield and I saw the barrel jump as the bullet tore into the soft metal jacket. That should put the gun out of action in short order.

"Here they come," I heard Jimmy yell.

I kept my sights on the German position. I could hear the men climbing into the crater as a German helmet appeared just above the trench top. I sighted on the helmet and fired. The helmet jerked, telling me the man had taken the bullet to the head. Losing a machine gun crew member and the water jacket should take them out of the fight for now.

Sliding down and turning around, I saw Private Woods passing out canteens. Right next to him was Father Mike, also carrying canteens and grinning at me.

"Good day, David."

Covered with dust and dirt, I saw he was not wearing a helmet, only his field cap.

"Padre."

He slid over to me, handing me a canteen.

"You look thirsty."

I had a drink.

"Thanks for coming," I said handing the canteen back to him.

"You were firing that rifle," he said.

Not wanting to discuss it, I just nodded.

"Corporal, I believe the machine gun is out of action. I think we can get these men out of here," I called to Jimmy.

"Right," Gallagher said and he got up and moved to the far side of the crater.

It took two hours with several bearer trips to get all of the wounded back to our lines. We left the bodies in the crater, as the Germans had begun rifle fire from the far end of their trench. At some point the dead would be recovered.

I wasn't going to risk any of our boys after what they had been through.

"Jimmy, your lads did very well out there. I'm proud of all of you."

"It's good when we can bring 'em in like that."

Major Bennett was standing at the end of the communication trench as I headed back to the bivouac.

"I'm sorry about James," he said. "He was a fine man."

"He was, he surely was."

I followed Jimmy's crew as we walked back to the bivouac. No one was talking much, the day having taken its toll on all of us. I was covering the same ground that James walked on his way to his aid station this morning. Walking to his death.

What in the hell is wrong with me? I can't let myself be overcome by either events or casualties. It is part of war and I am a soldier. I proved that today by killing an enemy soldier. Again, I caught myself. Don't dwell on any of this. Just take care of the men and do your duty.

But I was kidding myself. These things were having an impact on me. Perhaps I didn't realize how much.

One thing that I would have to deal with is that right now, I don't feel anything about having shot the German soldier. Not horror, not sadness, not remorse, nothing.

Back at the medical tents, I saw that last few wounded were being carried to an ambulance. With the sun starting to set, another day on the killing ground was drawing to a close.

At the far side of the tent, Private Sullivan sat quietly by himself. The bandage was still around his head and eyes and his hands were clasped as if he was praying. I stood there and realized this was what I was here for, take care of these men.

"Dan," I called to Corporal Jennings, who was standing outside.

"Yes, doctor."

"We'll be keeping Private Sullivan here for now. I'll need a liter of Ringer's solution, a sterile bowl, and a 10cc syringe with a number 18 needle. Get the private on the table and prepped for cleaning his eyes again."

Opening the storage chest, I found the cocaine hydrochloride powder. Mixing 50 grams of the powder with one liter of Ringers would produce a 5% solution for anesthesia of his eyes.

Dripping the solution at the far side of the eye, would numb the eye while simultaneously cleaning the eye of any debris left from earlier. I hoped that would then allow me to determine if there was any additional damage.

One hour later both eyes were cleansed. Unfortunately, it appeared there might be foreign matter imbedded in the scelera of the right eye. I bandaged both eyes and directed Dan to get the private a bed for the night. Realizing my concentration and coordination were compromised, I knew it was time to stop.

Jonesy had been assisting me the entire day and now sat on a crate going through his medical bag.

"Are you as tired as I am.

A corporal I recognized, but couldn't remember his name ran up to me.

"Captain, the colonel wants to see you in his tent."

Perhaps the war was about to be over for me. He had every right to court martial me for disobeying his order. But I did what was demanded medically. That was good enough for me.

"Captain McFadden, you heard me call you in the trench, didn't you?"

"Yes, sir, I did."

"But you felt that the medical needs of the men took priority over the orders of your battalion commander who could not possibly understand the medical situation."

"I was focused on the needs of the wounded men. I know that I should have obeyed your order. But I was devastated after what had happened to James Edwards."

"Yes, that was terrible."

He was quiet for a long thirty seconds.

"Doctor, the difference between a decoration and a court martial is often a very thin line. You walked that line today. But what you did was a remarkably brave thing and likely saved the lives of those men. For that reason, I am recommending you for the Distinguished Service Cross. However, in the future, I would ask that you comply with my orders, I almost always have a good reason for issuing them. Like trying to keep my senior medical officer alive for the remainder of the war."

Returning to my dugout, I closed the tent flap and quickly poured a drink. Looking at James' bed and his gear I felt angry. Then I remembered the German I'd killed. What was the difference? One German, one Englishman. Two more casualties and for what?

Despite being up since before dawn and downing two glasses of scotch, sleep was not coming. Unusual for me. I wondered if it was shooting the German. I didn't think it bothered me, but maybe I was fooling myself. But the more I thought about it, the less it concerned me. Maybe that was it, the fact that I didn't seem to care about it was disturbing me. I had always considered myself a moral man and a Christian. Thou shall not kill was a commandment from the Lord. I hadn't thought of it at any time until now. Was I a fake? Had all of my religious instruction been only a hollow façade?

The hell with it. I need the sleep, and I don't need any more scotch. I reached over to my medical bag, found a tin of morphine tablets and put one in my mouth.

The next day, the battalion stood down to rest and recover. Just as well, the cumulative effect of the past weeks has hollowed out what had been a rebuilt unit after the first part of the Somme.

I actually felt good having gotten a decent night's sleep. The loss of James was still painful, but I understood it was my duty to press on. It was an easy decision, I would move Glen Rossi to the aid station. While I would miss his expertise during operations, I knew Dan Jennings could handle most routine procedures. Glen had demonstrated his ability with front line medicine and the men would be in good hands. I'd make Jonesy his medical orderly, which put Glen in good hands. After two years including many surgeries, I doubt if there was a better qualified medical orderly on the Western Front. I would miss having him at my side, but I knew Dan Jennings would be able to cover as both our anesthetist and assistant.

Near mid-day, while finishing my report on the loss of James, I looked up to see Father Mike coming down the path. He always seemed to be on a mission, his jaw leading the way, followed by those piercing eyes.

"Hello padre."

"David, how are you?"

"As you would expect after losing James."

He sat down opposite me.

"A terrible thing, terrible."

He was right, what else was there to say?

"You're angry?" he asked.

I thought about it. Was I angry? Yes, of course. But it was more than that. The war had become a continual slaughter of soldiers on both sides. But no one seemed to care. Both sides fielded more lethal weapons, more men died and nothing changed. Some of the front line trenches were in the same location they were two years ago. Good Lord, how long could this continue. For two years the allies had fed hundreds of thousands of men into the fight with no appreciable change in the balance. What would it take to finally enable either side to prevail?

"It's the senselessness of it all. The madness just continues. Perhaps we have to kill every German to finally stop this insanity."

"It looked like that's what you were doing yesterday, David."

"What do you mean?"

"I saw you firing a rifle at the Germans."

"I did. The bastard was firing at my orderly bringing water to wounded men. And I'd do it again."

"David, by regulation you're a non-combatant."

"So was James."

"David..."

"None of this matters, padre. We do what we have to do. If that means shooting a German, so be it."

I was angry, but it was a type of anger that I had only known lately. Suddenly I felt a fury inside me. I wanted to slap Gallagher. It was his type of business as usual that would allow this war to go on forever.

The padre stood up, put on his cap.

"Take care of yourself, David. This war has a habit of tearing men apart."

I watched him walk up the path.

"Padre, wait."

I caught up with Father Mike.

"I'm sorry. James' death is difficult for me."

His eyes told me that he understood, but he was quiet.

"Give me some time. I'm not a Catholic, but I think I need to make a confession."

"David, I am here to talk with you. As a priest or a friend."

He held out his hand and I took it.

"Thank you, my friend."

Back in my tent, I found my medical bag and took two morphine tablets. I would get on my bed and just relax.

I woke to someone shaking my arm.

"Wakee, wakee, doctor."

Glen Rossi was leaning over me, peering down like he was inspecting a corpse.

"Good Lord, Glen, I was taking a nap. What's going on?"

"We knew you needed some rest, but we truly do need some direction out here."

My head was fuzzy.

"What time is it?"

"0915 actually. I checked on you at 1600 yesterday and you were fast asleep. So I decided to let you sleep."

"Thanks. I took a little help for the sleep."

"Seemed that way to me. But it worked and you didn't miss anything important. Now, how about we drop by the mess for some strong coffee."

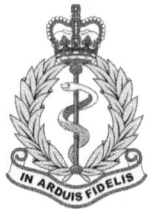

Chapter Twenty-Nine

"...the rat population seems to thrive during the winter months."

Gueudecourt France
December 1916

The bloodletting continued through September and October as the British army conducted three minor offensives against the German trench lines. The result was similar to the entire Somme offensive, small changes in control of territory and massive casualties on both sides. It was ironic that I now felt a greater animosity toward the British high command than I did toward the German troops. While we dealt with upper class generals, the Boche had their own Prussian aristocracy with the same disregard for the lives of their troops. At what point would the armies mutiny and put all the generals to the sword?

Reports out of Russia told of mass desertions following the revolt of February. Would that idea receive support from the armies on the Western Front? The French certainly have been decimated, Verdun being perhaps the bloodiest battle the world has even seen. I didn't sense a mutinous attitude among the troops, but I also thought that was something that could change quickly.

November turned cold, wet and miserable. It was difficult for all, but one result was a final end to the ongoing Somme offensive. In December the weather turned even more inclement. The war slowed almost to a stop as both sides tried to survive the frigid temperatures. Frozen water did help with the muddy trenches, but the effect on the men was horrendous. Apart from the frostbite, the increase in trench foot and respiratory ailments was staggering. Men on guard duty were at the mercy of the wind and frigid temperatures. While it had not happened to our battalion, word of men dying while on watch have come from down the line. With three more months before we could hope for a change in weather, I didn't know how we were going to keep the men fit enough to continue the war in the spring. I had found that I could stay relaxed as we dealt with the on going problems of supply and the cold. A good night's sleep was becoming a regular event and I was thankful.

Our casualties now were the result of poor food, hostile conditions, lice and a host of ailments including influenza, tuberculosis, dysentery, typhus and pneumonia, to name a few. The ongoing battle to provide clean water was even more challenging with the freezing conditions. Attempts at showering became infrequent with the expected misery of dirty bodies and dirty clothes. Despite the presence of many more dogs in the trenches, the rat population seemed to thrive during the winter months. The danger of rat bite fever and Tularemia was always present, the rats getting more and more aggressive as their food supply dwindled. Reports have come in that the increased rains have uncovered shallow graves from the recent battles and the rats have been seen feasting on the cadavers. It is difficult to imagine a more disgusting and depressing situation.

Our little group held up well. Rand Bernard has proved to be a trooper as Glen Rossi has. When anyone gets down, the others rally to their aid. Dan Jennings in his steady quiet manner is always there to deal with any problem. And Jonesy has become a truly irreplaceable member of the team. Who would have thought a young dispatch rider would have become an accomplished medical orderly and surgical assistant. Corey Timmons received his promotion to sergeant and no man was ever more deserving.

Glen Rossi also proved to be a superb scrounger. His time at the field hospital had given him an insight into and several good connections with the pharmaceutical providers. He was able to get us plentiful quantities of eucalyptus oil. I had thought that prevention might cut down on the cases of pneumonia and bronchitis.

The Royal Engineers built a treatment hut for our inhalation therapy. Working with the company commanders we began to be proactive, bringing soldiers in for therapy at the first sign of respiratory problems. It also gave us a chance to check their feet, issue them with new socks and foot powder. A small thing, but the dividends were spectacular. Our loss of soldiers sent away to field hospitals for respiratory problems plummeted. The instances of trench foot almost disappeared. It seemed we were winning small victories. God knows we had lost enough.

"Come in doctor."

The battalion commander was sitting at a camp desk, several papers in front of him.

I saluted and sat down on the offered seat.

"What can I do for you?"

"Sir, if operations would permit, I would like to take a week's leave and go to Boulogne."

"Boulogne?"

"My wife is a nurse at the hospital, a Red Cross nurse."

"I heard about her time with the battalion, rather unusual."

"The forward based surgical unit is still a good idea in my opinion, perhaps someday."

"Indeed, it seems to have merit in my estimation. In any case, the next two weeks will be quiet, assuming our German friends don't launch a major offensive. You need time off, it's clear you're tired. Go on, take your leave and get some rest."

An odd comment I thought. Did I appear tired?

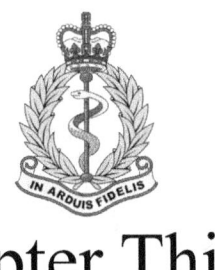

Chapter Thirty

"Doctor, I am desperately short on surgeons."

The Arras – Boulogne Road
24 December 1916

The ability to travel was impacted by the weather, but thankfully not by the availability of vehicles. What a change in the last two years, Where the war of 1914 seemed to be a horse drawn battle, by 1916, the automotive might of France and England had filled the roads of France with every manner of truck and automobile. I was able to catch rides with ease on the main road to Boulogne from Arras.

Finding myself in a Peerless 3 ton supply truck, I settled back on what should be only a four to five hour drive, putting us into . The truck was assigned to a supply company and my driver was a wiry private who hailed from Manchester. His name was Adamson and he had been in France for over a year.

"Have you been to Boulogne before?" I asked once we were on our way."

"Couple of times, normally I make the Le Havre run."

"Do you know where the 14th General Hospital is in town?"

He thought for a long minute.

"I think so. If I'm right, we pass it on the way to the depot. It used to be a big hotel, the Splendid if I recall."

"Good," I said, the journey now looking more promising.

"You a doctor, right?"

"That's right."

I had taken a pill to relax for the trip and his question made me think. I was a doctor. But not the doctor that arrived in France in 1914. Growing up, I watched my father live the life of an established physician, dealing with the daily ailments of life. The occasional death or accident seeming to be the only events that broke the very routine passage of time. Now I was dealing with a never ceasing nightmare of death and injury. The wounds I saw would terrify the most experienced doctors in London. Did that make me a better doctor or just one who knew how horribly the human body could be injured? I remember the initial shock of those first days. Now the devastating injuries all blend together.

The noise and jostling of the road seemed to fade and I pulled my great coat tighter, drifting off.

"There's the hospital, thought this was it."

The driver had pulled to the side of the road which ran by a curved driveway up to what looked like a main entrance. I could see large letters on the tap of the three story building that said "SPLENDID".

"Thanks, private," I said getting out and retrieving my case from behind the seat. The sun was starting to set, and I guessed it was almost 1800. A large civilian car was parked in the driveway, and an attendant stood at the double doors.

The man looked at me, nodded and pulled one of the doors open. Inside there were a number of chairs arranged along the entryway which led to a large double-wide desk elevated on a platform that served as a barrier. Two nurses sat at the desk, which I assume was where admittances were processed. They both looked up as I approached, their expressions showing curiosity.

My French was good enough to make simple conversation and discuss some medical issues. I told them I was looking for a nurse who worked in the hospital for the British Red Cross. The older of two got up, asking me to wait.

She returned with a much older nurse, in a uniform very different from the two younger nurses.

"I am the duty matron," she said in accented English. "Can I help you?"

"I am looking for Kathleen Su, I mean McFadden, from the British Red Cross."

"A moment, please."

She looked through a notebook on the desk.

"Nurse McFadden is on duty in our receiving ward, Ward Three."

"May I go there?"

The matron looked me over.

"You're a doctor?"

"I am, but I'm also her husband."

The matron smiled and waved to follow her.

Ward Three was in the rear of the main building on the second floor. It was clear as we walked through the corridors, the hospital was overflowing with patients. Many soldiers, still in uniforms soiled from the battlefield were on temporary cots in the hallway. Without a major offensive, how did this happen? Why weren't the overflow patients sent to other hospitals or evacuated to England? But this was not my problem, seeing Kathleen was all that mattered to me.

The ward was narrow with tightly packed beds on each wall running the entire length of a long wing of the building. There were at least sixty beds, all which appeared occupied. Looking down the ward, I saw only two nurses. Then I recognized her at the far end.

"Thank you," I said, not waiting for an answer.

Kathleen was tending to a patient, bending over the soldier with what looked like pills, while holding a water glass. I watched her gently put the pills into his open mouth, noting both his hands were covered with bandages. She gave him a drink, then set the glass down.

"Well done, nurse."

She turned her head briefly, turned back then turned full toward me.

"David," she said, and we embraced.

In that moment I was happy, very happy. In the last months her memory, her being, had faded slightly for me. Now I held her and we kissed. I'm sure there were regulations against public displays of affection, but we didn't care, and I don't think any of the patients who might have been paying attention cared either.

"I missed you, dear one," I said.

"And I you, my love."

"We can spend Christmas together."

"Our first Christmas as a family," she said, with a warm smile.

"We will make it very special, I promise."

"Nurse!"

I looked down the row of beds, a patient had his hand in the air.

Kathleen turned to see to the man.

The demands of war do not end because it is Christmas.

Confirming that Kathleen would be relieved at midnight, I promised to return after getting settled somewhere. She told me getting any time off would be very difficult. They were short staffed and had been working twelve hours on, twelve hours off for the last several months. While short on staff, they clearly weren't short on patients.

At the main entrance, I noticed a full colonel of the RAMC reading a notebook, open on the admitting desk.

"Excuse me, sir."

Looking up, he looked at me, then smiled.

"What can I do for you, captain?"

"Sir, I'm looking for the senior British medical officer."

"You have found him, sir. Doctor Pinkerton. What can I do for you?"

As I began to relate my situation, he held up his hand and asked me to follow him. His office was down the main corridor, and he ushered me in.

"Please, have a seat."

He was a tall man, and rather slim. He had a head of pure white hair and a magnificent mustache, also totally white.

"Doctor," he said, "It is Christmas eve, and I think I would like a drink. Would you join me?"

"Yes, sir, thank you."

"Scotch?"

"Yes, sir."

He poured two glasses, handed me one and sat down behind his desk.

"To your health," he said, raising his glass.

"And to yours," I replied.

He smiled and took a drink. He seemed tired to me, but perhaps it was just his age, which I guessed was near 60.

"What brings you to our hospital on Christmas eve? You said you were on leave."

"To see my wife. She's a Red Cross nurse at the hospital."

"Ah, McFadden, I recognize the name. Where are you assigned?"

"The Highland Light Infantry."

"Really?"

"Yes, sir. I'm the senior medical officer for the Second Battalion."

"So, you've seen some action?"

I relayed a brief summary of the last two years with the Second.

"You've seen quite a lot it seems."

"Too much."

Over a second drink, my experience with our forward surgical team came up.

"A forward surgical team? How were you able to get a surgeon up to the front?"

"I am a surgeon, sir."

"Indeed. Where did you train?"

"King's College Hospital, under Doctor Cheyne."

"Sir William, my that is something. Did you finish the course?"

"Yes, sir, took the MRCS just prior to going on active service."

"We have a Watson Cheyne trained surgeon assigned as a battalion MO?"

"A long affiliation with the regiment. Father was the MO in the Boer War."

"I see, rather unusual."

We sat for a moment, each looking at their drink.

"Doctor, I am desperately short on surgeons. The truth is men are dying because of it. There won't be a major offensive for several months. If I was able to have you attached to the hospital for a period of time, would you be willing?"

The idea had not occurred to me. But if the battalion was not going to be involved in any major actions, and with the winter now fully in place, actions should be limited. The idea of spending time with Kathleen was almost too much to consider.

"Sir, if my battalion commander agrees, I would certainly do what I can to help at the hospital."

We discussed how we might arrange this, and we agreed I would return to the battalion at the end of my leave and make the request of Colonel Prescott. This was quite the turn of events, but I found myself quite happy the more I considered the opportunity. While I had been practicing surgery for the last two years, I had missed the intense pace and complications of a major operating theatre. Rand and Glen Rossi would be quite capable of carrying on with the current medical operations. The proximity of Boulogne was another positive factor, I could be back with the battalion in a day. I told myself this might not work for any number of reasons, but it was worth raising the question.

At midnight, I made my way to the ward, noting that for a hospital at night, there was a great deal of activity in the corridors. The work of nurses in wartime never let up and the incredible flow of wounded to the major field hospitals like Rouen and Boulogne never ceased.

Kathleen was helping a patient drink water when I arrived. Walking quietly to her side, I realized her patient had lost both legs and one arm. The terrible toll on his body had completely missed his face and other than a very light beard, he looked perfectly composed although his color was clearly pale.

"Thanks, miss," he said, his voice faint.

"You are quite welcome, James. Now you need your rest."

She adjusted his covers and stepped back, smoothing one edge of the bed.

"Will you be able to leave?" I asked, not seeing any nurses other than the second nurse from earlier.

"Elizabeth will be here shortly. I will need to do my turn over, but that won't take too long."

"We have a room at the Folkestone. Colonel Pinkerton has a car for us also."

Kathleen looked surprised.

"You met the Colonel?"

"We had quite the conversation, I will tell you about it later."

The Folkestone lived up to its reputation as having the best service in Boulogne when they provided a midnight supper of soup, bread and wine for Kathleen and myself in a dining room lit by only candles.

I told her of the plan to use me as an adjunct surgeon if the battalion would agree. She stood up from her place at the table, walked around to me and hugged me so tightly, I thought I would burst. It was delightful and reminded me that newlyweds are very special creatures.

"David, we're so short on staff with three of the nurses on leave in England, I'm afraid I won't have any time off from my rotation."

"Well, if the colonel agrees, why don't I start my work here and then at the end of the week, I will make the trek back to the battalion."

She let me know that we could talk about that later as she took my hand and led me toward the main staircase upstairs.

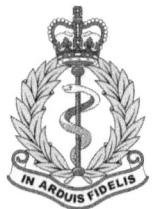

Chapter Thirty-One

"Sir, I just wish the generals spent more time on the battle line."

General Hospital Number 14
Boulogne
6 January 1917

The battalion was scheduled to return to the rear as part of the rest and re-equip plan the second week of January. Colonel Prescott did not expect any major activity until at least March. He was most agreeable to my proposal and even mentioned that Doctor Rossi seemed well capable of standing in for me.

Officially General Hospital Number 14 was capable of handling one thousand patients. I was told that on several occasions during the Somme offensive the actual number of casualties reached over 1500. While the flow of casualties had slowed significantly, the work of recovery and rehabilitation never ceased. My primary work would involve follow on surgery that took place to further remove foreign bodies, normally shrapnel, repair areas that had been hastily treated in a lifesaving effort and the most difficult, the amputation of limbs that had finally been required due to the lack of healing or and thankfully less often gangrene.

Colonel Pinkerton had been a wonder, finding a cottage only a mile from the hospital we were able to rent for as long as I was in Boulogne. The cottage came with a maid/housekeeper/cook by the name of Jeanne

Dupuis. A widow since 1914, she spoke quite passable English, a great comfort as my French was marginal at best.

I was looking forward to operating in a fully staffed and equipped operating theatre. It would be similar I hoped to what I had trained on in London. Swinging by Kathleen's ward, I wanted to see her before I started my first day.

"Good morning, my lady."

Kathleen looked up from a patient as she was finishing with an intravenous drip.

"David, good morning."

"Busy I see."

She helped me step away from the patient's side.

"Ringer's, but it seems like we are just going through the motions."

"What do you mean?"

"The young private has an abdominal wound. Most likely the doctors will avoid surgery and the result will be poor."

Abdominal wounds have been traditionally the most lethal. Wounds tended to become infected, either from external factors or damage to the bowel.

I checked the patient tag and saw the man had been wounded late yesterday. The patient data was limited as he had only been on the ward for two hours. But my evaluation was that surgery now could perhaps beat the infection.

"Thomas Wolf, private, Royal Hampshire Regiment."

Looking down I could see the young man had his eyes open. Abdominal wounds could go bad so quickly, his only chance was surgery now.

"Hello soldier, I'm Doctor McFadden. How are you feeling?"

"Not bad, just cold and sore."

"We can take care of both, you rest easy."

"Kathleen, how do surgery orders generate here?"

"Once the lads are here, a staff doctor will come through and evaluate each man, putting them on the list for surgery if he feels it is warranted."

"Has anyone seen Private Wolf?"

She shook her head.

"It often takes some time for the evaluation," she said quietly.

I knew timeliness could be the difference between living and dying.

"Colonel, I saw a soldier in Ward Three a few minutes ago. He arrived late last night and has not been evaluated. I believe he needs surgery right now if he is to have a chance of surviving."

Pinkerton was sitting at his desk, a steaming cup of coffee next to his blotter.

"Type of injury?"

"Abdominal. Small entry wound. I don't think it was a bullet, shrapnel more likely."

He looked at me hard.

"You're telling me he should have been evaluated sooner."

"Colonel, I would not think to tell you how to run this hospital. But I will tell you as a doctor who has seen wounded men for two years, he needs surgery."

"Then let's go take care of him, doctor."

I found out when Pinkerton spoke, people acted. In twenty minutes, we were over at the former casino, now serving as the location for a group of operating theatres and a recovery ward.

As we walked over, he let me know his surgeons wore full gowns during surgery and he encouraged masks and gloves but did not require them. They only used ether for anesthesia, would use spinal anesthesia when called for and there was a portable x-ray machine, although it was currently broken.

"I will assist you, doctor. We only have two anesthetists so the assisting surgeon will fill in when needed."

Outside the theatres a very modern washing area allowed me to completely wash my hand and arms with a carbolic soap. I had trained without gloves and felt I needed the tactile feel during procedures. Doctor Pinkerton pulled on a mask, which was my signal to do the same.

We were led to theatre number two, located in what appeared to be a former salon. The lighting was superb, better than I was used to in London.

Two nurses were also gowned, both wearing masks.

"Nurses, if you would?" Doctor Pinkerton said as we approached the operating table.

The first, taller nurse said, "I'm Nurse Adkins, from the Red Cross."

"Your first name, please?"

"Betty, doctor."

"Thank you, Betty."

"I'm Katherine Luce, doctor, Imperial Nursing Service."

"Katherine, thank you. My name is David McFadden. I ask that you listen carefully to any requests and do not hesitate to speak up if you see a problem. Understood?"

They both acknowledged my directions.

"Private Wolf is from the Royal Hampshires and needs a bit of work to get back to fighting trim. Right, Thomas?"

The young man nodded with a slight smile.

Doctor Pinkerton held the Clover Ether Inhaler.

"Thomas, just breath normally."

I felt comfortable as I watched the senior physician monitor young Wolf. As effective as ether was, the patient must be watched closely for respiration, blood pressure, pulse and any muscular activity.

Wolf coughed several times, not unusual with ether.

In about eight minutes, Doctor Pinkerton looked up from the patient and said, "We're ready."

Relaxed, his chest moving rhythmically, Private Wolf now needed our very best work.

"Let us proceed," I said.

The nurses removed the drape from his midsection, the area having already been thoroughly swabbed with iodine. The entry wound had been uncovered, showing a one inch gash

"For the record, the entry wound is located in the lower right quadrant, three inches inferior and three inches lateral to the umbilicus, overlying the right iliac region."

Knowing that metal, bullets or shell fragments could take bizarre paths in the body, I chose to make my incision across the entry wound itself.

The nurses were obviously experienced as they smoothly passed Metzenbaum scissors, forceps and retractors to me. I was relieved there was no evidence of severe hemorrhage, but clearly there was some type of compromise under the small intestine.

"I need to flush with Dakin's, please."

Nurse Luce used a large syringe to begin irrigating the incision area.

"Nurse Atkins, please be ready with sponges to remove the liquid."

She approached the opposite side of the table with several sterile sponges on wooden sticks.

"Work to one side, Betty, I'll be looking for the bleeder."

The tear in the small intestine was evident as I carefully moved the bowel for inspection. The damage was minor, and I knew I could suture it successfully, lowering the probability of infection.

Using catgut sutures I repaired the tear in short order, allowing me to continue looking for more damage, the shell fragment or the source of the bleeding.

"Hold the Dakin's, please."

"Betty, clear as much fluid as you can, I need to find the bleeder."

It was clear the source of the bleeding was from behind the small intestine. There are several potential culprits, and I needed to narrow it down. The midline looked to be the most likely location, telling me the superior mesenteric artery could be the source. A gentle examination confirmed a nick in the artery. Again, luck was with young Wolf, the damage was not severe and the bleeding was not fatal.

After suturing the damage, I continued my search for any other problems. That examination revealed a small piece of jagged metal, perhaps one half inch in length. I removed the metal, making one last check for any bleeding.

Another full flush with Dakin's and it was time to close the incision. My plan was to leave two rubber drains each at the low point of the incision curve.

The final sutures went in at the two hour point. Now the challenge of bringing the patient out of the ether induced unconsciousness.

Nurse Luce rolled in an oxygen tank with the face mask already attached. The use of oxygen to assist the patient to clear the ether from his system was becoming more prevalent over the last several years. It reduced the often seen complications of vomiting , nausea, and shivering. Two blankets were placed over the private just before he was moved to the recovery room.

I took off my mask and said, "Ladies, thank you for assistance. I believe that the procedure was done in time, and he has a much better than average of recovering from his wounds."

As they began post procedure clean up, Doctor Pinkerton said, "I think a cup of coffee is in order, doctor. Would you join me?"

Over steaming coffee in his office, we went over several items, nothing of great note, more like a review.

"What would you say to taking the job of initial evaluation on the receiving ward? It strikes me that your field experience would make you likely the most qualified physician in the hospital."

The logic made sense to me. I was used to initial exams of wounded, it was part and parcel of what a battalion doctor does daily. I also liked the idea of working with Kathleen daily.

"I would look forward to taking over those duties. But would I be still in the surgical rotation?"

"Most assuredly. I think it would be the perfect arrangement."

"Private Wolf likely will recover. But there are so many that arrive here days after being wounded. What do you see as a remedy to the problem?"

"It's simply the logistic challenge. Many of our positions have three trench lines, those trenches may be two thousand yards apart, connected by comm trenches. Moving a patient through that maze is the job of the stretcher bearers. During a major action, there are simply too many wounded and too few bearers. And most of our wounded in those circumstances are well beyond our forward trench, requiring the bearers to find them and then carry them across shell pitted terrain, often under fire."

"Quite a challenge for such junior soldiers."

"We do train them to make basic determinations of survivability. These men take their jobs very seriously, but there is only so much they can do."

The colonel nodded.

"Once they get to the ambulance stations," I continued, "our transportation capability is quickly overwhelmed. Failure to get to a casualty clearing station will then delay transfer to the second line of ambulance or train transport. So, by the time they reach a field hospital it can be days from being wounded. I guess we're lucky that we don't use horse drawn wagons like we did in 1914."

"How do we fix the problem?"

"Moving patient care closer to the front," I said.

"Explain."

I went over our forward surgical team experience. He asked all of the right questions, but stopped me in my tracks when he noted, "You put those nurses in danger, didn't you."

"I think you'll find that most nurses are willing to face those dangers in order to care for the lads. We have to use every resource we can and nurses make a difference doctors can't compete with."

"How so?"

"We don't have the time to devote to follow up care that, in my opinion, is critical for the survival of many patients. I spent time in a ward in Rouen and saw it firsthand. The young soldiers are completely different when interacting with nurses compared to doctors. There is a humanity that is palpable. Maybe it's a fall back to the care of a mother, but many times I saw a soldier respond to the care of a nurse that would never have happened with a doctor or even an orderly. There's just some kind of magic and we need to take advantage of it."

"Doctor, it's clear your time with the troops has given you an entirely different viewpoint than many other and more senior physicians. I wish more doctors had your experience on the battle line."

I laughed.

"Sir, I just wish the generals spent more time on the battle line."

Doctor Charles Pinkerton looked back at me without comment. But it was clear to me he understood my point.

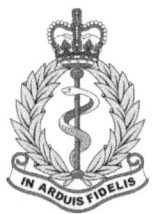

Chapter Thirty-Two

"But, I will die tomorrow."

General Hospital Number 14
Boulogne
March 1917

Ultimately, I spent nine weeks at the hospital. Despite the long hours, I felt more rested every day as I was able to take care of soldiers and work with Kathleen on the ward. I often thought my idea we could work together after the war had some merit, now I knew it was fact.

But the never ending grind of the war caught up with me the day Jonesy arrived with a note from Colonel Prescott requesting my return to the battalion.

"Is something in the works?"

"No one knows for sure, but ammunition stores are being delivered along with cases of Mills Bombs."

The spring offensive was starting to take shape.

"How are our ranks? Did we get replacements?"

"Criminy, yes. Every company is fully manned, and the new ones seem too young to shave."

"We've seen it before, Ryan."

"Aye, that we have."

The letter from the colonel asked that I return by the end of the week. I appreciated the leeway, several cases of mine would do with a few more days of observation. I would also have at least three more days with Kathleen.

"Would you like me to request your permanent assignment to the hospital? God knows your contributions in such a short time had a very positive effect on both the morale and efficiency. Perhaps with a title such as "Medical Director?"

Doctor Pinkerton was the type of senior physician I had always wanted to work for. His invitation was powerful. I would be able to affect the care of many more men than at the battalion. But that was the problem. The Highland Light Infantry was my regiment and always would be. To leave Jonesy, Glen Rossi and Dan Jennings on their own was something I wasn't ready to do.

"Sir, I made a commitment to my regiment and I must honor that. My time here has been a God's send, both personally and professionally. When this war is over, I would be honored to work with you."

The colonel smiled.

"Doctor, I will hold you to that."

Returning to the cottage together was unusual for us. The conflicting schedule and emergencies resulted in our arrivals and departures around the clock. Today, the stars fell in line and I would be able to tell Kathleen I was going back to the front.

She had been quiet during the taxi ride from the hospital. The long shifts took their toll and quiet seemed to rejuvenate her after a long day. I thought a nice dinner, several glasses of wine and I would be ready to tell her and hopefully she would be ready to accept it.

Jeanne Dupuis' cooking had been a true pleasure after eating army rations. In fact, my general distaste for French cuisine was cured as I was introduced to the rustic cooking of the common French kitchen. Never having tried cassoulet, I was stunned when she combined fresh vegetables, white beans and sausage in a dish that demonstrated what the right combination of herbs and sauce could do. I would truly miss her cooking when I returned to the battalion.

"Hello, Jeanne."

The aroma from the kitchen told me she had been working her magic again.

Kathleen brushed past me toward the bedroom and I went into the kitchen to confirm Jeanne was making her cassoulet.

"Hello, David."

"You made my favorite dish, thank you."

"I know that you like it and I was able to find a wonderful sausage in the market today. May I pour you a glass of wine?"

"Yes, please. It has been a long day."

She smiled.

"All of your days and Kathleen's too are long, too long."

"Jeanne, I am going back to the front at the end of the week. It will be hard on Kathleen, but I know you will take good care of her."

Her eyes showed that she understood the danger.

"I will take care of her," Jeanne said, handing me a glass of wine. "Some day this horrible war will end."

I lifted my glass to her.

"To that day, madame."

"Would you like a glass of wine, Kathleen?"

She had brushed her hair and stood at the kitchen door.

"Not tonight, David, I am feeling a bit under the weather."

"When did that start?"

Kathleen walked through the kitchen to the small dining room.

"This morning," she said, sitting down at the table.

She put her hand to her mouth and coughed.

The cough sounded very deep, not like her at all.

I walked over and felt her face.

"I think you are running a fever."

She nodded.

"I do feel flushed."

"Is your throat sore?"

"Scratchy."

"Let me check your throat."

She coughed again, that same deep sound.

"I be right back," I said.

With the illumination of my torch, I was certain I was seeing the beginning of diphtheria. Last winter I had seen too many cases and the lining of Kathleen's throat was displaying the telltale grey tinge. Early detection and injection of the diphtheria anti-toxin had almost universally prevented fatalities in the battalion. But it was a tough slog for several days, fall on one's back and generally miserable.

"My dear, I am going to the hospital. I'll return with the diphtheria anti-toxin and get you on the path to recovery."

"There were several cases in the ward this week, that must have done it."

"I am prescribing at least five days of bed rest under the care of Jeanne."

"What about her?"

"I'll bring a dose for her. If she starts showing any symptoms, give her the shot."

"Can't you do that?"

I told her of the letter ordering me to return to the battalion.

"I don't leave until the end of the week, so I'll be able to take care of you until then. If you need any more help, contact Doctor Pinkerton, he'll make sure you are taken care of."

"He's quite a nice man," she said, not even complaining of my leaving. Her two years in this war have made her wise in the way of the military. We both knew the separation would be hard, but we both would also be very busy and time does fly when busy.

Three days passed and it was time to head back. Jonesy had enjoyed four days of good food, wine and sleep and couldn't stop smiling. The early dose of anti-toxin resulted in a mild case for Kathleen, which could not have made me happier. In addition, Jeanne was showing no signs of the illness when I finally left the cottage.

I had become used to living indoors over the last nine weeks and as I watched the rain pelt the windshield the reality of wet feet and mud came back all too quickly.

The battalion was five miles behind the main trench lines just southwest of Brielen. It was clear when I arrived, the battalion was back up to strength. Rows of tents for the men, plus larger tents for messing and administration made the camp look quite formidable.

I reported to the colonel and thanked him for the opportunity.

"Doctor, you've paid your dues. It was the least the battalion could do for you. I'm surprised the rear echelon brass didn't put their hooks into you permanently."

I laughed.

"They made a quite attractive offer, actually."

"You say?"

"Medical director, working for one of the best doctors I've ever met."

"And you came back to work for a right bastard like myself."

With a grin, I replied, "Indeed, sir, I couldn't help myself."

Prescott laughed as I had never heard. He was quite different from Lieutenant Colonel Abernathy, but he was still a man I would follow with confidence.

"The reason I needed you back was an operation which we'll be undertaking in seven days. This is part of a plan to put the army in a better position to commence the spring offensive."

He opened a map on his desk and pointed to the depictions of the current trench lines, ours and theirs.

"The Ypres salient. A thorn in our side for two years. The initial phase will be to take the salient and then move deeper into the enemy's heavy support systems, the rail system and supply depots. In order to do that, we have been ordered to attack this strong point, located on this ridge. From there, we will be able to direct fire on the right flank of the Germans."

"Strong point?"

"Reinforced trenches with multiple machine gun positions, in some cases protected by concrete."

"A difficult objective to this layman."

"Doctor, you are quite right. I'm afraid the potential for casualties is very high."

The war had returned with a vengeance.

"Sir, I have a request."

"Go ahead."

"I would like to have Private Jones promoted to corporal. He is a superb medical orderly and had taken on greater responsibility continually. He now has over two years in the battalion and has been in every fight we've had."

"That, doctor, is an easy decision. Make sure the sergeant major gets the paperwork done and he can put on the stripes straight away,"

The promotion was a small thing, but very important to me.

"Medical director, you don't say."

Glen Rossi welcomed me back with a short libation. He said it was to warm me up after the cold and wet journey from Boulogne.

"And how is your lovely wife?"

"Until several days ago, she couldn't have been better. The time we spent working in the receiving ward was wonderful. She's a remarkably effective nurse as you well know. In the ward, she was truly taking care of those boys. Unfortunately, she just came down with diphtheria."

"Damnation."

"I was able to get her the anti-toxin straight away and think she'll have a relatively easy time of it."

I told him about Jeanne Dupuis, her cooking and caring for Kathleen.

"I'm sure she'll be fine," Glen said.

"In the meantime, it appears we have a challenge coming up in seven days."

"That's what I've been hearing in the mess, but nothing specific."

In a quick overview of the operation, I told him we needed to be ready for heavy casualties. My conviction on rapid surgery had become even stronger at Boulogne watching the men arrive who should have been treated earlier.

"I want to set up our surgical team right at the push off point. We also need to make sure Jimmy Chesney has enough bearers. At least eight teams."

"Aye, I'll make sure."

"Over the next seven days, I want to brief those teams. Four hours a day with you, me, Dan Jennings, Corey Timmons and Jonesy. While we're doing that, Rand can work on supplies and make sure we're ready to go. Have the new orderly, Sutton, work with Rand. That was they can get to know each other and Sutton will be with Rand in his aid station. Also, let's make medical pouches for each of the bearers, not just the team leader. More bandages and morphine out among the lads can only help."

"Good idea."

"And Glen, I want at least one pistol on each team. Jonesy can work on that. Sergeant Seaton owes me a big favor and he can get the weapons. I'll talk to Jonesy. I don't want this to get any notice, so minimal fuss, but I don't want those men out in No Man's Land without some ability to defend themselves from the random German."

I remembered the chaos during and after an attack. You never knew who you might encounter.

Jonesy had been surprised when I told him of his promotion, but it was clear he was very proud. He had been so important to me over the last two years and was now a remarkably competent medical practitioner. His future after the war would be well served if he took up medicine. I would keep him thinking about the possibilities.

I was able to borrow a motorcycle and sidecar for my next task. I wanted to find the best location for our forward surgery, not wanting to wait until the day of the attack. Thankfully the map I had been given by the colonel was well annotated. With Jonesy and I deciphering the directions, we found the jump off area.

The main trench was currently manned by a battalion of the Welsh Fusiliers. The troops were more than happy to show us the layout of the main trench and the attached communication trenches. I could sense they were relieved they would be withdrawn prior to the attack. My questions about the German positions told me that these lads wanted no part of attacking the complex. Along the front, there were areas that had changed hands over the last two years. Not so here. The enemy has been improving these positions since 1914. I can only imagine the difficulty they'll present to our battalion. I located a dugout currently was being used as officer's quarters. The area was larger than most, well equipped with duckboards to keep the mud to a minimum on the floors. A generator provided electric lighting, which was a welcome surprise. I would make it clear to the colonel this area would be for surgery.

On the way back to our bivouac, we were stopped by military police, directing a very large convoy down the main road. We realized it would take some time before the convoy was clear and Jonesy found a copse of trees for us to wait.

We took off our goggles and sat down on a fallen log. I noticed my young protégé looked tired. I knew he'd just turned twenty, but he had the face of someone in their mid-thirties.

"Are you feeling well?" I asked.

"Fine, why'd ya ask?"

"You look tired."

He laughed.

"Hell, we all look tired. It's the damn war, nothing else."

"Have you heard anything from Alice?"

He shook his head.

"Did you write her?"

"I did. Nothing back."

"Like you said, it's the war. Never can count on the post."

"Aye, maybe."

"Are you ready for what's coming?"

"The attack?"

I nodded.

"I'm sick of the wounds, the dead lads, the dirt, filth and everything about it."

Was I losing my best orderly?

"But we can take care of them, and we're damn good at it."

"Ryan, other than finding Kathleen, running into you at Le Havre may have been the best thing I've done during this war."

He turned and looked at me, grinning.

"I guess I'm lucky that bloke slashed me."

Three days before the attack was scheduled to commence, the battalion loaded onto trucks and made the ten mile trip across the front to our new positions. There was speculation as to why trucks had been provided. A ten mile move would normally be done on foot with some of the equipment loaded on trucks or carts. Were the brass treating the shock troops special? Did they expect major casualties like the Somme. The mood among the lads was grim and the normal banter was missing. Too many veterans knew what was coming.

Following the offload and set up, I was in the admin tent when I heard men outside.

Father Mike entered the tent, his expression concerned.

"David, I need your help."

"What's wrong?"

"Corporal Hewes is outside. He came to me and told me he couldn't do it anymore."

"Can't do what?"

"Fight, make himself charge the German lines."

I could only sigh. There was nothing to do, men had been shot for deserting or failing to attack the enemy.

"I suspect most men in the battalion would prefer not to attack tomorrow."

"David, please take a look at him."

"Very well, have him come in."

The corporal walked in, although it was more of a shuffle.

"Sit down Hewes."

He was perhaps 22 or 23, average height, a bit slender with a totally blank expression on his face.

"Do you feel well, corporal?"

He nodded.

"Be more specific," I asked him.

"Aye, well....sir."

His voice was quiet, with little annunciation. Was this an act?

"Chaplain Gallagher tells me that you are having problems with doing your job."

"Yes..sir."

"Are you afraid of dying?"

"Yes, sir. I am."

I stared at him expecting him to act nervous, but his face remained blank.

"Don't you think everyone fears dying?"

"Aye, sir. But I will die tomorrow."

"Why do you say that?"

"It's my time."

"If you're ordered to attack, will you advance with your men?"

"I don't know."

"You know that cowardice can result in a court martial and possibly the death penalty?"

He nodded slightly.

"Does that scare you?"

"I don't know what to do."

Nor did I. The mind is a difficult thing, and I have no great insight. It seems Corporal Hewes is serious, but do I refer him to the provosts?

"Corporal, open your shirt."

He looked at me with surprise, the first indication of any emotion. Slowly he unbuttoned his tunic.

"That's fine," I said when he had four buttons open.

I put my stethoscope in my ears and leaned forward to listen to his chest.

Sitting back, I said, "Corporal, I am diagnosing you with pleurisy. It is clear you can't go back to duty. So, I will keep you here at the admin tent. If you are not better by tomorrow evening, I may perform a thoracentesis to drain any excess liquid from your lungs. Understood?"

He looked at me for a moment, then said, "Yes, sir."

Perhaps he just needed some time. I could certainly give him that. If he eventually refused to fight, I would have to let the lawyers deal with it.

By evening, I felt the medical staff was trained, ready and equipped. But my experience now told me once the whistles were blown, chaos would return, and we would have to adapt.

Glen, Rand and I sat in my tent, a bottle of Glenlivet open on my side table. We decided a final tactical review was in order to make sure all details had been addressed in our plan. While a "tactical review" was tongue in cheek. I did want to go over the surgical plan one more time. The key would be to ensure we moved casualties needing surgery to the dugout from the aid stations as quickly as possible. My challenge would be to evaluate the men sent by Rand and Glen to decide the order of surgery. Both Corey and Jonesy would assist me, and I was counting on the sergeant to direct the stretcher bearers for the best result.

I took a drink, marveling at the quality of the scotch. There were many things done right in Scotland, but distilling scotch must be regarded as one of the best. Never did I imagine my consumption of spirits would rise to this level, but as we say, it's the war. Since my time at Boulogne, my use of morphine had dropped significantly, and I intended to keep it that way.

As our evening session broke up, a messenger from the battalion commander handed me a note.

"Please stop by and see me as soon as you can. P"

"Come in, doctor."

Prescott was sitting on a folding stool, several official looking documents on his lap.

"I just received this from a motorcycle messenger. I was quite surprised as the use of motorcycles is almost always critical tactical orders from the brass."

He handed me what looked like a plain envelope with "Battalion Commander, Highland Light Infantry" printed on the outside. Inside I found a piece of stationary with "Doctor Charles C. Pinkerton" embossed on the top.

David,

I am sorry to have to tell you that Kathleen has taken a turn for the worse. Despite the timely administration of anti-toxin, her throat has become quite swollen. I was forced to perform a tracheotomy to allow her to breath comfortably. At this point, she is relatively comfortable with a low grade fever. I feel that the next 24 hours are going to be critical. Your presence could make all the difference.

Sincerely,

Charles Pinkerton

A tracheotomy, I was stunned, not something normally done, Doctor Pinkerton must have been very concerned. Thank God a surgeon of his experience was there for Kathleen. But if her throat was that swollen, the disease must have progressed much more aggressively than I had expected. I was sure the early dosing with anti-toxin would have resulted in a mild period of discomfort and rapid recovery. So much for my diagnostician skills. Damn.

"Doctor, you look like it's bad news."

"My wife has taken a turn for the worse in Boulogne."

"I'm sorry to hear that, David. Is there anything I can do?"

I could ask for leave. It was only a five hour trip. I could be there in the morning. But the coming events of tomorrow morning brought me back to reality. My duty was here, taking care of the men of the Highland Light Infantry. But what about my duty to Kathleen? If my presence could make a difference, how could I not be there?

"Sir, I need to go to Boulogne. But I will not ask for leave until after the attack tomorrow, and see how things go."

The battalion commander nodded and said, "We can talk tomorrow."

I stepped out of his tent, the rain now coming down in sheets. This was going to be a nightmare for the men trying to advance in what will be a wet and sodden battlefield. My thoughts, dark already, took a turn for the worse.

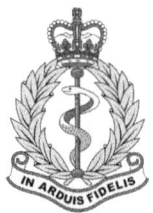

Chapter Thirty-Three

"A good man if there ever was, but in this war it didn't matter."

Forward British trench
Near St. Julian
31 July 1917

Just before 0400, the artillery barrage began. Having been in France for two years, I thought I knew what an artillery barrage sounded and felt like. My previous experience did not prepare me for what took place in the early hours of the 31st of July. Thank the Lord it only lasted for a short time before we heard the whistles telling our men to advance.

Jonesy, Corey and I moved out into the main trench from our dugout to watch the troops move to the ladders and pull themselves up and over into the unknown. There was little talk other than a few smart remarks which were obviously nervous men trying to show the expected bravado of the infantry, several of the men looked at me, their expressions tense as they pushed forward.

Many of the men were new recruits and could not know what awaited them. But for the veterans, it always put me in awe to watch them go forward, knowing the horrors they would encounter. I thought of the tens of thousands of young men who had gone before and to their deaths. Again, the lunacy was clear to me, but it was what it was.

When the men were past, the three of us returned to our dugout, or surgery if you will. Formerly housing several officers of the Welsh Fusiliers, the only major change needed was the installation of an operating table. The Royal Engineers accommodated our request and now we were ready to take casualties. Three former bunks would allow us to have a pre-op area.

So, we were ready. Glen Rossi and Dan Jennings were in their aid station about one hundred yards northwest up the trench. Rand and Sutton the same distance to the southeast. We had our area covered, now God hope we wouldn't be needed. But I was not a fool.

As expected, the sound of machine guns now replaced the artillery barrage. If I listened carefully, I could tell they were German Maxims. The barrage, as always it seemed, never destroyed the German machine guns, waiting to tear our men to pieces once again.

The first bearer team was Jimmy Chesney's.

From outside the dugout, he called, "Doc, here's a patient."

Stepping outside, the bearer team, other than Jimmy, were on their knees, resting from carrying their wounded soldier.

"Doc, you were the closest aid station."

I knelt down and saw the patient had been hit in his right shoulder, perhaps several bullets judging by the blood and torn tunic.

"Good decision, Jimmy, get him inside."

Under the electric lights, the blood was evident, oozing from under the thick bandage, held in place with a cloth cord.

"Put the stretcher on the table," I directed.

The young soldier groaned as the stretcher was slid onto the table. The stretcher bearers left the dugout, their stretcher now serving as an impromptu operating table.

Immediately, Jonesy began cutting his equipment straps. He had lost a great deal of blood, his tunic soaked.

"What's your name, soldier?" I asked.

His reply sounded like "Turner" but with the noise level, I couldn't be sure.

Cutting the bandage off, I saw what remained of his shoulder. In addition to the soft tissue damage, white bone fragments protruded from the wound. One of the bullets must have shattered the upper humerus. The only hope for this young man was to get him to a CCS as soon as possible.

"Ryan, I need to pack the wound and secure it for transport. Jimmy, I need you lads to get him to the pickup point as fast as possible, understood?"

"Aye, sir."

I leaned over the private, with a doubled over gauze pad. The blood was oozing and I hoped a strong pressure padding would hold until he got to an appropriate facility.

Slamming down on the patient, I felt a tremendous force on my back, shoving me down and forward. My feet were off the floor and my body was falling head first. A sharp pain in my side and total darkness were the sum of my senses. Was I dead? I didn't think so, so we must have been hit by an artillery shell.

My left arm was immobilized, perhaps by soil from the overhead or the support beams. Reaching out with my right arm, I could feel the underside of the operating table. I seemed to be partially wrapped around it but could not move either leg. I coughed, the dust heavy in my little chamber. Thank God I was able to breathe, but for how long? Would anyone know what had happened? My face was resting on a metal surface that I realized was the waste can from under the operating table.

"Jonesy, Corey," I called, hoping they were in the open.

Reaching back up toward my right leg, I tried to find the patient. He had been face up on the table, and might have taken the brunt of the cave in face first, which did not bode well.

"Can anyone hear me?"

No response. I couldn't hear anything. Shouldn't I be able to hear shovels if they were digging?

Trying again to move my legs, the pain in my side made me gasp. Running my hand over the painful area, I could not detect any open wound. Internal injuries, perhaps cracked ribs. A complication certainly, but if I wasn't found, it didn't matter.

Try to ease the breathing and listen for any sign of rescue. In the midst of a battle, the silence was unnerving, but it would help me hear any digging, I was sure. Relaxing my head against my metal pillow, I tried to think if there was anything else I could do?

"Help," I yelled, the pain lancing into my side.

The only connection to the rest of the world remained the vibrations of the earth as artillery shells continued to impact our lines. Deep in the distance I could hear the attendant rumble of the explosions. Was everyone around me dead? No one might know I lay here. The morbid thought occurred to me that this might be my grave, Lord no.

Did I hear something? I listened with all my concentration. A scraping sound. Could that be a shovel?

"Help, help, over here," I screamed, hoping they could hear me.

Suddenly I felt a tug on my left ankle. Then the feel of a hand around my lower leg. Noise of men yelling, dirt cascading down from above and then light. Thank the Lord.

"Hold on, doc."

Hands were around both legs and I felt the dirt pinning me to the operating table being shoveled away.

"Careful now," came a voice that sounded like Jimmy Chesney.

In a minute hands were around my shoulders and pulling me out of the remains of our operating area. I saw the body of our patient, a large wood splinter driven through his chest. Killed on the operating table, my God, will the horror never end.

Brushing dirt from my face, I looked around for Jonesy or Corey.

"Jimmy, did you find Ryan or Corey?"

"Jonesy's around the corner," he replied, pointing to the bend in the trench.

Getting to my feet, I was still a bit unsteady, but able to walk down the trench, using the wall for support. Rounding the turn, I saw Jonesy slumped against a canvass tarp, his eyes closed.

"Ryan, are you all right?"

He opened his eyes and slowly turned his head. The vacant stare in his eyes said concussion to me.

I knelt down and quickly checked for any bleeding or signs of trauma.

"Mother of God," he said slowly, "My head is coming apart."

I noticed both pupils were equal and reactive, a good sign.

"Do you remember what happened?"

He shook his head.

"I want you to just sit here. Lay back and close your eyes. I need to check on Corey."

"Right," he said softly and closed his eyes.

Jimmy and his crew were still digging when I got back to the dugout. It seemed Corey was back by the sleeping area when Jonesy and I were working on the young soldier. Was he still there?

"Jimmy, have you dug over by that black beam?"

"Na yet," he said.

"He might be there. Do you have another shovel?" I asked, then knew my side would keep me from helping anyone.

"Come on," Jimmy called to his bearers.

Twenty minutes later, Jimmy found Corey's body, completed encased in soil from the dugout's overhead. While there are no good ways to be killed, suffocating under a ton of dirt, unable to move or cry out, is truly horrible. We moved his body to a ground cloth. I began cleaning the dirt from his face, mouth and nose. It seemed obscene to have a man's life ended by dirt. In ten minutes we had him cleaned up and covered with another ground cloth. A good man if there ever was, but in this war it didn't matter.

I returned up the trench and sat down next to Jonesy. My friend's eyes were closed. We had been through so much over the past two years. A few minutes to catch my breath, then I would get Jonesy to an aid station. The dark clouds were moving across the sky, and I felt the first drops of rain on my face.

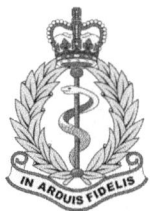

Chapter Thirty-Four

"My duty is here, and I will stay as long as we are engaged with the enemy."

Forward Aid Station
Near St. Julian
31 July 1917

By the time we neared Glen Rossi's aid station the rain was beating down. The ground, already wet from previous rains was rapidly turning into mud. If the duckboards in the trench were in good repair, making progress had been reasonable, but in some areas the water was already over the wood. I was afraid if this rain continued it would repeat what we saw last fall, a sodden terrain unfriendly to friend or enemy.

Jimmy and I helped Jonesy down the trench, his gait slightly unstable but steady. He had been quiet as we moved east toward the aid station. The trenches were mostly empty except for the defensive machine gun emplacements and a skeleton infantry force to patrol the area. The ongoing din of machine gun and rifle shots rose and fell along with the explosions of German minenwerfers.

Ahead a dugout opening appeared, a chance to get out of the rain and rest for a minute. The deserted space did have a single electric light on, allowing us to see it was a berthing area of sorts. We helped Jonesy sit down in a wood camp chair. Jimmy and I sat on ammunition boxes, removing our helmets.

"Ryan, how are you?" I asked.

Jonesy had his head in his hands, elbows resting on his knees.

"Fucking head," he said.

We had already given him two morphine tablets and I wanted to wait until we reached the aid station before we gave him anymore.

"We're almost there, just rest for now."

Jimmy sat quietly, the powerful body relaxed and quiet as usual. A unique man, he could be the loud corporal with his teams if needed, but he seemed to enjoy quiet more. I thought of Corey Timmons, very much the same. Left to his own, he enjoyed the quiet, but could take whatever action was needed to complete his job. Then it struck me.

"Jimmy, with Corey dead, I need a new medical orderly. You've been handling bandages and wounded men for two years. Now you would be with the doctors taking care of more medical duties. I've listened to your lectures, and you know a great deal about this business already. What say you?"

"Who would take care of our bearers?" he asked.

"Who would you recommend?"

He thought for a moment.

"Private Langdon would be my choice."

"Then Private Langdon it is."

The aid station was past busy, and we found an out of the way spot for Jonesy, gave him another morphine tablet and began to help Glen and his new orderly. I mentioned to Glen that Jimmy would be our new orderly and he was pleased.

"A good lad," he said, "Must have some Canadian blood."

My side was uncomfortable, but I was able to work around it, paying close attention to my movement. Jimmy was a God send, being another set of hands for me.

The constant rain made for a more than miserable day as we tried to keep up with the casualties. Wounds were by far from machine gun fire, not the normal shrapnel we were used to seeing. While some shrapnel wounds were often minor based on the size of the fragment, there were no minor bullet wounds.

The DWM MG08 was the preferred heavy machine gun of the German army. It fired an 8mm bullet at a rate of over 400 rounds per minute. The damage of a bullet impact was significant, and many soldiers were hit by more than one round. In the chest abdomen area, the rates of fatality were high. Hitting and arm or leg might often necessitate an amputation. Blood loss was often the immediate danger, and it was not unusual for death to occur before the wounded man could even be carried to the aid station. Our stretcher bearers made all the difference with their use of tourniquets and pressure bandages. Today everything was complicated by the massive amounts of mud, dirt and debris from the battlefield. But that was the way of things.

By midday, the processing of wounded was steady. Despite the number of casualties, the presence of myself and Jimmy made a great difference. I checked on Jonesy several times and he was resting albeit uncomfortably.

A German artillery attack at our main trench line and rear support areas opened up a half past noon. The impacting artillery shells coupled with the ongoing deluge of rain produced a hellish afternoon. Then we heard the gongs, signaling a gas attack. Christ.

I stuck my head out to see if there were any obvious gas clouds in the area, which thankfully confirmed none around the aid station. Gas masks were pulled out of cases and I had one of the walking wounded take up a lookout station.

The Germans had been using phosgene for the most part, but our intelligence reported the enemy now had mustard gas as well. Phosgene raised hell with the lungs, pulmonary edema being the major cause of death. Mustard gas was reported to burn the skin and could also wreak havoc if inhaled. We would keep at it, with masks on those who could tolerate it and pray for those who could not.

Over the afternoon, we saw no evidence of gas in our area and were able to treat and pass casualties along unhampered.

"Ryan, it's back to the camp with you," I finally said at almost 7:00. The flow of casualties had slowed and with the sun going down, the recovery of wounded would be minimal. I needed to find the battalion commander and pass along my report on the wounded.

"Jimmy, make your way to Lieutenant Bernard and get his report. Grab four of the bearers and then meet me back in camp as soon as you can."

He nodded, put on his helmet and headed out.

It took almost an hour to make our way back to camp. As luck would have, I was able to find out where Lieutenant Colonel Prescott had his headquarters. Our main admin tent was still in good order, and I set about getting Jonesy some food and then into his bed roll. One advantage of the RAMC was the provision for sleeping bed rolls. The line troops were not as lucky and had to rely on simple ground sheets and blankets.

"How are you, my friend?"

Jonesy smiled.

"Can you get me a new head?"

"No, but I can help you sleep tonight."

I gave him two morphine tablets cut into four.

"One now and one anytime you wake up if you can't go back to sleep."

He put one in his mouth and closed his eyes.

"Sleep well," I said as I stepped out of the tent.

"Doc, over here."

It was Jimmy.

"Here's Doc Bernard's note," he said, handing me a folded piece of brown wrapping paper.

"The only thing he had that was dry," Jimmy explained.

I read the note by lantern and saw their day had been much like ours. The battalion had taken over 90 casualties processed through the two aid stations. No count of the missing and dead at this point and if experience has taught me anything, there were the same number of men laying in the mud in No Man's Land. Some of those men were wounded and would be spending a painful and lonely night as the rain continued to beat down.

An hour later, I delivered my report to the battalion commander. He accepted the news gravely. With a total wounded and missing close to two hundred, the battalion was down to seven hundred effectives.

"Orders for tomorrow, sir?" I asked.

"Nothing formal as of now. Our lads advanced about one thousand yards and are holding the main German defensive trench opposite our lines. If I'm right, the enemy will counterattack when the sun comes up. Right now, our job is to hold what we have taken."

"For now," I said, "I'll count on the bearers to carry the wounded across No Man's Land to the aid stations. The mud is making transport to the Casualty Clearing Station at Lingier difficult, but the ambulances have been able to get through."

He nodded.

"What about your wife?"

I was surprised that with the events of the day, he remembered my problem this late in the day.

"Sir, I am confident that Doctor Pinkerton will provide the best care possible. My duty is here, and I will stay as long as we are engaged with the enemy."

"Thank you, doctor."

Back at camp, I saw Jonesy was resting quietly. My surprise was the presence of Corporal Hewes, sitting in the tent, almost on watch.

Sitting down next to the young man I asked, "How are you feeling, corporal?"

He didn't answer at first.

"Better, sir," he said after a moment.

"I see."

The corporal was fully kitted out and it was 2:00 in the morning. Was that a message to me?

"Are you ready to go back to your company."

He hesitated, then said, "I – I think so."

While he did not sound like his doubts were gone, he did convey he was ready to go. Perhaps a little more time to settle down.

"Corporal Hewes, I have a job for you before that."

"Sir?"

"Corporal Jones has, at the very least, a severe concussion and possibly a hairline fracture of the skull. I could keep him here and watch for symptoms to develop or I could get him to somewhere he can be treated."

"Aye, sir."

"Normally he would be sent to a casualty clearing station and treated there or sent on to a hospital. I'm going to bypass the CCS. I want you to escort him to General Hospital Number 14 in Boulogne. Once there, you will report to the hospital commander, Colonel Pinkerton. I will have a letter for you to deliver to him which will explain everything he needs to know. I want you to spend two days at the hospital and then return here to report on Jonesy's condition. Can you do that?"

"Yes, sir. I'll take care of him, you can trust me."

"I have no doubt, corporal."

Jimmy Chesney entered the tent, and I could hear other men behind him, hopefully the bearers.

"Did the lads get some rest?"

"Aye."

"I'll pack up several medical bags with supplies and then we, along with the bearers leading the way, will catch up with the forward troops. I know there will be wounded men who have chosen to stay at the front, and we can take care of them. If the German are true to form, they will likely counterattack. Do you have your pistol with you?"

"I do."

"Can you hit anything with it?" I smiled.

He grinned back at me.

"If I'm close enough."

"That may not be a problem."

Jonesy had reacted to the noise and was now sitting on his bedroll.

"How's the head?"

He blinked twice and nodded.

"Better. Sleep helped."

I told him of our plan.

"I don't need to go to the hospital, I'll be fine."

"I want Doctor Pinkerton to look at you just to be safe. But I also need you to check on Kathleen."

Jonesy knew what was going on and the look in his eyes told me he understood.

"Corporal Hewes will go along with you to handle any problems. I hope you both can be back here in two or three days. Doctor Pinkerton will likely send a letter to me about Kathleen."

"I understand, doc."

"Thank you, my friend."

Jimmy, his bearers and I made our way back to the battalion's primary trench and I was able to locate Captain Barry Ashton, who commanded the security troops. He showed me his current understanding of the forward progress by the battalion. They were currently occupying a stretch of the German's main defensive trench and some parts of the next trench about 100 yards further into the enemy terrain. Despite the darkness, I felt we would have no problem finding our lads, and setting up an aid station.

"Have the Germans tried to retake their trenches?" I asked the young officer.

"So far, they haven't, but we expect them to try. Our artillery will start a barrage at first light to discourage any attempt."

"Thank you, Barry."

"Keep your head down, David. There has been activity all night long. The German's have not taken this lightly."

The sarcasm in his voice made me smile. While I had no knowledge of any other enemy, the Germans have proven to be a brutal and incessant foe. The list of casualties certainly makes that point.

Private Snowden, the team leader for this group of bearers had been across No Man's Land recently and took the lead of our group as we moved through the first line of our own barbed wire. Our immediate concern was the possibility of flares over us, highlighting our position. Everyone knew that on the lighting on any airborne flare, dropping to the ground and taking cover was the only acceptable action. We would remain motionless until the flare burned out, then strike out again.

Five minutes after leaving our trench line, we were covered with mud up to our knees. The torn up terrain and torrential downpours now presently a landscape that was mud, mud and more mud. Large artillery craters were to be avoided, the depth of water in some over five feet. Any remnants of prior gas attacks also would leave poisonous debris behind. This was all inhabited by a remarkable number of rats, who seemed immune to the dangers of warfare and nourished by the bodies of the dead.

The ignition of an airborne flare sent us all down on our stomachs, the whitish light flashing across the landscape. In the distance I heard a German machine gun begin firing, but not in our direction. It told me that they were not sleeping tonight and as we closed to our positions, it would get more dangerous.

As the flare burned out, I heard Jimmy, who was up ahead with Snowden call out, "Up you go."

I felt the mud clinging to my tunic and could only try to pull some of the larger pieces off with my hands. I knew the mud would also be attached to our equipment bags and the two stretchers we were bringing with us.

Ahead an explosion briefly lit up the sky, the noise echoing across the fields. I suspected they were the German minenwerfers, which our boys called "minnies." The short range mortar was lethal for anyone in the open and had caused heavy casualties over the past year.

Two more flares interrupted our progress, but did not cause any fire directed our way. I expect the Germans were still getting used to the new landscape and had not established good fields of fire yet. If the line remained static for any time, they would have this area covered, there was no doubt in my mind.

"Halt, identify yourself."

"Medical party," I heard Jimmy respond.

He exchanged passwords and we were cleared to proceed.

As we climbed down into the trench, I could see most of the men were at least trying to sleep, ground cloths serving as improvised shelters. I saw a sergeant I recognized from B Company.

"Sergeant, is your company commander here?"

"Aye, sir. Follow me, I'll take you to him."

Captain Herbert Turley, Herb to his friends was looking at a map in one of the German dugouts. I was impressed with the construction of the shelter. Large beams interspersed with logs seemed to provide a remarkable level of protection. Although it was lit by candles, I could see electric lights hanging from the ceiling. All the comforts of home.

"Hello, doc. Didn't expect to see you up here."

"Good evening, Herb, I was out for an evening walk and just thought I would swing by to say hello."

We shook hands.

"I brought equipment to set up an aid station and take care of any wounded you may still have here."

"We were able to get a large number of men back to our trenches, but we do have a dugout with our wounded at the end of the next trench."

"I'll examine them right now. We have one team of stretcher bearers, but we brought another stretcher if you have any men you could spare."

"Sergeant, pull four men from first platoon. David, will your bearers teach them the ropes?"

"They will and lead them back to our aid stations."

An explosion in the distance made us both flinch, the concussion just perceptible through the dugout opening.

"Never will get used to those infernal things," Herb said.

"What are your casualties?"

He looked tired.

"80 men killed, wounded or missing."

The battalion had finally gotten back to strength and in one day, decimated again. How does an army achieve a victory if all it does is bleed itself dry?

"I'm sorry, Herb. It all seems so futile sometimes."

"You will not get an argument from me."

"I'll go look at your lads."

Jimmy and I carried our muddy medical bags to the next trench and found the wounded men. Half of them were sitting up, bandages in evidence. One of the men was smoking a cigarette while the others had their eyes closed.

"I'm Doctor McFadden, what's your name soldier?"

The man grimaced and said, "Brooks, Private Brooks."

"Just relax, I'll see you in a minute, after I check some of your mates."

Of the four men lying flat, one was dead. The other three had painful but not life threatening wounds.

Private Brooks sat with his back toward the wall, his left leg stretched out on the sleeping platform. A large bandage covered his left thigh, which I began carefully cutting off.

His pants had been cut away and the left side of his thigh showed the effect of a massive impact. The bruising was hard to believe and in several areas the skin had ruptured, leading to blood loss. The other most obvious problem was his broken femur. The break was not compound but presented distended flesh on the inside of his thigh. The pain must be terrible.

I noticed his wound card tied around his right wrist. It noted morphine pills given three hours ago.

"I'm going to inject your thigh with morphine. It will help with the pain."

I saw almost an immediate effect on the private. He relaxed against the wall. We needed to get him flat.

"Jimmy, give me a hand here."

The two of us carefully moved him to a horizontal position, making sure to immobilize his thigh.

"Jimmy, let the bearer team know they have to bring back a Thomas Splint so we can move the private back to our lines."

The remainder of the men were not seriously wounded, and we made sure their wounds were cleaned and bandaged well and left them to rest. It was almost sunrise when we were able to sit down and get our equipment ready for what might come with the new day.

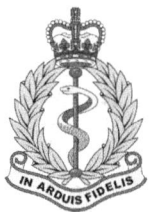

Chapter Thirty-Five

"I see you managed to get yourself bayoneted."

Main German Trench
Near Zonnebekke
1 August 1917

The faint light of dawn was accentuated by the first shells landing in a German barrage of their captured trench system. The intensity increased as heavier guns were added to the gun line. The inherent strength of the German defenses became apparent as we took shelter in the protected dugout. The wounded that could move, found as much cover within the dugout as they could, moving into corners and cubby holes.

While the opening to the dugout was only the size of a double door, some debris from the shell impacts fell into our space, despite the canvas barriers hanging down from the top of the opening.

Was this the beginning of a German attack? Herb expected one, but hadn't made any predictions when that might happen. The Germans could be attacking right now.

"Jimmy, we need to be ready for a German attack."

The big man looked at me for a moment then said, "Attack?"

"This artillery barrage could be the beginning."

"What should we do?" he asked.

We had seven wounded men who should be treated as non-combatants and taken prisoner if the Germans retook the trench. But I knew the chaos of an infantry battle was unpredictable. Would attacking troops recognize this was a medical dugout? We could try to mark it somehow and hope the Germans would respect our medical status. I also knew that both the British and Germans used grenades to deal with enemy trench dugouts. Would we get a grenade through the door before we could surrender?

"Make sure your pistol is loaded and ready. If the Germans show up, we will surrender, if possible, to protect the wounded men. But if things get out of control, be ready to defend these men."

He nodded.

"Right."

I just hope it doesn't come to that.

"Stand to…..Stand to!"

The universal call to be ready for battle echoed down the trench. I could hear movement in the walkway outside and put my head out to see the troopers rushing to station themselves along the wooden duckboards. The problem was obvious, the trench had been constructed to fight forward toward our lines. Now our men had to defend the trench from the backside where the fighting platforms were almost non-existent. Men were moving anything that might serve as a step up to the back wall of the trench. As they piled wooden boxes, steel drums and tarps at the base of the wall, German machine gun fire began to rake the top of the trench. Dirt, mud and rocks flew in all directions as the German fire blanketed the trench. All we could do was take cover until the fire ceased, knowing the German infantry would then attack.

Ducking back into the dugout I took time to stop by each of the wounded. All I could say was to stay steady and that the corporal and I were here to take care of them.

Jimmy and I took positions near the entrance to try and monitor what was happening. The problem for me was that I really couldn't see what was going on from inside the dugout.

"Stay here, I'm going to see what's happening."

Pushing to the open, the dim of machine gun and rifle fire left no doubt this was an attack. I had no idea what to expect and crouched down as the troopers returned German fire. The logs on the top of the trench wall provided some protection, but the continual machine gun fire was keeping our men's head below the trench line.

A burst of Maxim fire hit the log, and I saw one of the men fly back across the trench and hit the front wall, falling in a heap on the duckboards.

Jumping down I knelt next to him and rolled him over in the early morning light. The front of his face above the eyes was torn open, blood covering his eyes, which remained open. The poor man was dead, never knowing what hit him.

Suddenly the German machine gun fire dropped off and I heard whistles up and down the trench. A Vickers machine gun crew moved their weapon to a firing position in anticipation of the coming attack. The trench was well manned, and I saw the entrance to the dugout was not standing out in the reduced lighting. Perhaps that was the natural defense.

"Liquid fire!"

The cry from a man on the trench told me that the Germans were moving forward with their Flammenwerfer. The thought was frightening, if they made it to the trench, they could spray burning fuel into the trench, incinerating everything. I pulled my Webley.

The Vickers opened up, and despite the horrific roar of the gun, it gave me comfort we were defending ourselves. But I wasn't sure what to do. Sliding down the front wall of the trench, I went to the dugout entry and knelt down in a carved out area opposite the dugout. This was as good a place to defend the dugout as any.

"Jimmy," I called out, not sure he could hear over the din.

One of the canvas tarps was pulled aside and I saw Jimmy's face.

"The German's are attacking. Hold tight. I'll keep watch out here."

He nodded, holding up his pistol and then his face was gone.

I could see the orange light coming from the direction of the attack and realized it must be the liquid fire. I was scared and there was no reason to try and fool myself. Leaning back into the cut out, I held my Webley ready, waiting for the German soldiers to swarm over the trench top.

Our lads continued to return fire, the Vickers firing continuously. A bright flash made me think they had reached the trench, but the light was followed by a explosion. Had the German carrying the flame weapon been hit?

A German soldier appeared at the top of the trench. He fired his rifle and jumped forward, taking one of our boys down to the trench bottom. The two struggled just feet away from me, both fighting with their hands, having lost their rifles. The Brit fell backwards, and I saw the German pull a knife from his belt. He moved toward our lad, and I pulled the trigger. He turned sideways, now just seeing me and I fired again. The man collapsed.

I saw more Germans at the far end of the trench. Shots echoed off the walls of the trench and a grenade detonated. The struggle remained near the Vickers crew, and I saw the machine gunners in hand-to-hand battles with the enemy.

I stayed in place, my Webley ready. How long would this go on, and when does the fight end?

Behind me a heard a yell and turned to see two German soldiers, carrying rifles with bayonets. They were on me and all I could do was fire the Webley. The first man stumbled, my bullet hitting him in the chest.

I stood and stumbled back as the second soldier thrust his bayonet at me. Something caught my foot and I felt backwards as the man tore my left leg with the bayonet. We both fell to the ground and his head lay on my lower leg. Twisting I brought the Webley around and fired into his face.

His dead weight pinned me to the ground and I tried to pull myself free.

Looking up, I saw Jimmy's face.

He pulled the German off me and I realized the bayonet, attached to the rifle was still in my leg. Then the pain began.

"What do I do?" Jimmy asked.

I tried to answer and was short of breath, just able to say, "Hold.."

With my hand in the air, I just needed a moment.

In the distance I heard the Vickers firing, that was a good sign. Damn the pain, it shot up my side and into my gut. Had the bayonet hit my gut?

Slowly I got my breathing under control.

Gritting my teeth I said, "Watch out for Jerry."

Looking down, I saw the German rifle on the duckboards, the point of the bayonet having pierced my leg. The dead German lay on his side, thank God not on the rifle.

"Jimmy, go get a medical kit."

I would have him pull the bayonet out as straight as possible to prevent more damage. He could then pack the wound with gauze and bandage it. I could only hope there was not any damage to the main artery in the leg, in which case I would simply bleed to death.

"Here," Jimmy said laying the canvas bag next to the dead German.

"I need you to pull the rifle and bayonet out slowly and as straight as you can. Any twisting will do more damage to my leg." I gasped as pain ran up my leg and into my groin.

"Right," he said, getting down on his knees. He pulled a pack of gauze from the kit and lay it on my trousers.

He looked me straight in the eyes and asked, "Ready?"

I nodded.

Resting on my right elbow I watched him grasp the Mauser and with both hands begin to pull. For a moment the rifle did not move, then it pulled out several inches, prompting Jimmy to stop.

"Damn, damn, it slipped, sorry."

"No harm, just a steady pull. Go ahead."

The pain throbbed, but there were no shooting pains as the blade was slowly withdrawn.

I waited to see what would happen as it cleared the wound. Would there be a strong bleeder or just oozing?

With the bayonet withdrawn, Jimmy said nothing as he took a pair of scissors and cut open my trouser. He took a gauze pad and held it against the wound.

"Jimmy, you need to force the gauze into the wound, both the entry and exit."

"Right."

He cut the rest of the trouser leg off and reached for more gauze.

I felt the bandage being pushed into the exit wound. Once this was done, it was time for morphine.

Just before taking two pills, I had Jimmy fasten two pressure bandages to the two bayonet punctures. Thank God it appeared there was no compromise of the major arteries of the leg.

Jimmy and one of the walking wounded helped me into the dugout and lay me on one of the bunks. I drank some water and then drifted off.

I woke up to voices in the dugout.

"Let me take a look," I heard Glen Rossi say and then saw him leaning over me.

"I see you managed to get yourself bayoneted."

"Not my idea," I said, trying to smile.

He took my pulse, temperature and made a cursory body check.

"We brought two teams of bearers out and a Thomas Splint as you requested. Our intent is to move all of the wounded back to the aid station. Rand is setting up there now."

"Private Brooks is over against the wall. He needs the splint badly before he goes anywhere."

"David, we'll take care of it. Now let me take a look at your leg."

With the morphine having taken full effect, I lay in a fog as Glenn attended the other wounded and got them ready for moving back to our lines. My leg throbbed, but I was able to put it in the back of my mind. It is funny how the body can adjust to severe conditions and move on.

"Do you need anything?"

I opened my eyes to see Jimmy standing next to my bunk.

"A hot bath and stiff drink, if you please."

He smiled.

"I do have some fresh water."

"That actually sounds wonderful."

He gave me a cup and helped raise my head so I could drink.

"Thanks."

"How's the pain?"

"It's all right."

"It's a field hospital for you, I'm thinking."

Boulogne if I have any control I thought. A chance to see Kathleen. The thought made me feel good. Perhaps a good thing would come from a bad thing.

Two hours later, evacuation of the wounded began. I waited until they all had gone and Jimmy took charge of the last bearer team for the trip back across No Man's Land.

When we got back to our lines, Jimmy located one of the ambulances and we put Private Brooks and myself in for the trip to Boulogne. Some might say we were hijacking the system, but both of us needed hospitalization and there was no need to be processed through a casualty control station.

Just before we left, the battalion commander found me.

"Boulogne, right?"

"Yes, sir."

"Perhaps you asked that German to bayonet you so you could see your wife?"

He had a slight smile on his face.

"Sir, the thought never occurred to me."

His face became serious.

"Hand-to-hand combat with German assault troops?"

"There were eight wounded we had to protect."

"David, that was a hell of a brave thing to do. Corporal Chesney filled me in on the details."

"Sir, Chesney deserves promotion to sergeant. He has become one of the primary members of the medical department."

"I will take care of it. Now give me your best estimate on when we might get you back?"

"No idea. I have to find out how much damage that blade did to the leg. The other unknown is infection. I hope it bled enough to flush the wound, but only time will tell."

"Understood."

"Rossi and Bernard will take good care of the battalion until I do get back."

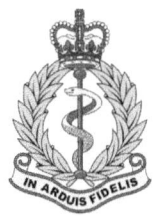

Chapter Thirty-Six

"Aren't we the pretty two?"

General Hospital Number 14
Boulogne
2 August 1917

Rain fell constantly during the seven hour journey north. The road was heavily traveled with trucks traveling both directions to and from the battle area. Our driver was an old hand, and the ride was as comfortable as one could imagine in the situation.

When we finally arrived at the hospital, it was close to 8:00 PM. I didn't recognize the attending nurse who directed our litters to Ward Three. It seemed the old system was still in place. It was good to be inside, the rain continuing to fall heavily in the night. I wondered where Jonesy would be and what was his final diagnosis?

The morphine was wearing off and I communicated that to the charge nurse when I was finally lifted onto the bed in the ward. A second nurse looked past the charge nurse. I recognized her, but could not remember her name.

"Doctor McFadden. I saw your name and notified Doctor Pinkerton. He should be along shortly."

"Thank you. I'm sorry I don't recall your name."

"Morris, Betty Morris."

"Thank you. Do you know how my wife is?"

"She is doing well. Doctor Pinkerton can give you all the information."

My spirits soared.

"David, it is good to see you, despite the circumstances."

"Colonel, this wasn't planned, but at least I will be here for Kathleen. What can you tell me?"

"The 24 hours after the tracheotomy were very concerning. But then she literally turned the corner. Temperature went down, lungs began to clear. She still has the tube inserted, but I expect to remove that in the morning if she continues to improve."

"Can I see her?"

He smiled.

"I expected no less. Let me check your leg and then we will put you in a wheelchair and take you down the hall to see her."

My impatience was tempered by my friendship with Doctor Pinkerton. He took thirty minutes to remove the bandages, check my leg, insert a drain at the entry point and lightly bandage the leg.

"Now off we go to see Kathleen. But you and I will meet in the operating theater in about an hour. I need to open the wound and ensure it is clean. I want a full flush with Carrel Dakin's and make sure there is no dead tissue. As you well know, time is of the essence."

He was right and I knew that was the only way to ensure I did not end up with gangrene and lose the leg. His skill as a surgeon was superb and I could not be in better hands.

Kathleen was in a small room with only two beds and she had the room to herself. I wondered if she would be asleep, it was after 10.

Her head was on a double pillow with side pillows to prevent her head moving from side to side. A blue bedspread covered her to her waist and her gown was tied open at her throat. I maneuvered the chair alongside the bed and saw her hands lay at her side. Her hair was covered with a type of scarf.

For a moment I just looked at her face. She seemed to be asleep, and I was willing to wake her to make sure she knew I was here for her.

I took her right hand carefully and held it, watching her face. At first there was no movement, then I saw her eyes open.

"Kathleen, it's David."

I squeezed her hand.

"I know you can't talk, but I'm here with Doctor Pinkerton and he told me that the tube will probably come out tomorrow. Then we can talk all we want."

What should I say about my wound? He had turned her head slightly and I pushed myself up with my good leg so she could see my face.

"I hurt my leg, but it's really nothing. But it means I will be able to spend time with you for a week or two. By then you should be fully recovered."

I saw her lips move and pulled myself up far enough to kiss her.

"I love you."

Her lips moved and she mouthed the words I love you.

Doctor Pinkerton leaned over.

"Kathleen, you need sleep and so does David. I will see you in the morning."

As we rolled back to Ward Three, I asked.

"Did you see my medical orderly, Corporal Jones?"

"I did. It was a very good decision to send him directly here. Our radiographic apparatus is working and confirmed a fracture of the skull in two places."

"What are your thoughts?"

"The traditional rest for now, but if the severe pain continues it may call for surgery. He seems confused at times, and I noticed some slurred speech."

Intracranial bleeding could be the problem and it is life threatening. Thank God I'm here for him.

An hour later I lay on the operating table. I recognized everyone standing around the theatre. Betty Adkins and Kathy Luce had assisted me on a number of surgeries. Doctor Phillip Layton was going to serve as anesthetist.

"Well, David, we brought in the first team for you. This will be very straightforward. We'll open the bayonet wound, ensure there are no issues or debris within. A thorough flush with Dakin's will be conducted. My intent is to not only leave the incision open, but also install a drain at the entry point. A light bandage will allow continued monitoring over the next week."

"Thank you all, I couldn't be in better hands. Doctor Pinkerton, I'm certainly ready to proceed."

I heard him tell Phil to begin.

"Breathe easy, David."

Phil placed the ether mask over my face.

I told myself to relax and began a steady rhythm with my inhalations. The normal time for the ether to take effect was ten minutes so I knew what to expect. The ether was raw on my throat, but not such that I needed to cough. I had seen patients vomit or cough during the administration of ether and only hoped I would not be one of those.

Firm hands were on my arms as I began to come out of the anesthetic. Several coughs helped to get me back with the real world, although my throat was now particularly sore.

I saw Betty standing over me, holding an oxygen mask.

"This will help," she said, putting the mask to my face.

The oxygen was cool and felt good on my throat.

"There were fabric bits in the wound," I heard her say. "But we saw nothing else of note. Doctor Pinkerton will be in to see you shortly."

After ten minutes of oxygen, she removed the mask.

"Feeling all right?"

I nodded. Often nausea is present after ether, but I felt nothing.

"Hello David."

I opened my eyes to see Doctor Pinkerton by my bedside.

"How are you feeling?"

"Still coming out of the anesthesia, but I am doing well."

"Everything went quite well. Some debris in the wound, but a solid flush took care of that."

"Muscular damage?"

"Always hard to tell until we close and give you a chance to rebuild your strength."

"Right."

"In any case, we both need sleep. I will take care of Kathleen later this morning and you will be able to talk with her."

"No concerns?"

"There is never any guarantee as you well know. But I feel very good that this will be left behind her as a bad memory. But with her husband at her side for probably a month, I suspect she will be focused on other things."

I smiled.

"Now, get some sleep."

"Doctor Pinkerton. I want to see Corporal Jones as soon as possible."

"I will have a wheelchair ready for you as soon as you feel up to it."

Betty Adkins helped me into wicker wheelchair, already fitted with an elevated platform which allowed me to rest my leg in the horizontal position. Insisting that she push me for the initial run, we made our way to Kathleen's room.

It was mid-morning and Betty let me know that Doctor Pinkerton had removed her tracheotomy tube earlier.

Kathleen sat propped up on several pillows, her hands in her lap and a smile on her face.

Neither of us said anything as Betty pushed me to the bedside and quietly left.

"You look wonderful," I said, meaning every word. She seemed so calm and someone had brushed her hair.

I took her hand and softly squeezed it.

When she spoke, her voice was soft, "I didn't know if we would ever see each other again."

"It was meant to be, don't you think?"

"You were wounded?"

I nodded.

"Doctor Pinkerton took care of it last night. All I have to do now is rest."

"It is so good to see you," she said putting her other hand on top of mine.

I did love her, more than I could have ever imagined.

Ryan was in Ward Four, a smaller ward with only a dozen beds. All were occupied and I immediately saw him in the second bed on the right.

His eyes were closed, and I gently shook his leg.

I watched him stir, then saw his left eye open, followed several seconds later by his right.

"How are you doing, my friend?"

He looked at me with a puzzled look on his face.

"My bloody head won't stop…stop hurtn'."

"I talked to the doctor, and he told me that you may need surgery."

"You're the doctor," he said squeezing his eyes closed.

"Jonesy, it's me, David McFadden."

Turning his head, he opened his eyes."

"Doc, what are you doing here?"

"Don't mind that, I am here, and we're going to get you taken care of."

Doctor Pinkerton must have known the reason for my visit. He had a viewing stand near his desk with a radiographic plate already mounted.

"How are you doing, David?"

"The pain is very manageable, thank you."

"I expected you wanted to consult on Corporal Jones."

"I was able to talk with him, and it is my opinion that there must be some level of intracranial bleeding to present the continuing level of pain along with his confusion and slurred speech."

"A reasonable conclusion," he replied. "The question is whether we wait for possible resolution or opt for surgery now. You and I both know the risks."

"Yes, sir. You certainly have more experience that I do on cases like this, but I don't think the chances of a natural resolution are very high."

The colonel went through the ritual of lighting his pipe.

"Shall we look at the radiography," he said.

I rolled myself over to the viewer while he turned on the illumination.

"We have three views here, anterior, posterior and lateral from both sides."

After examining each of the plates, it was clear my friend had a single fracture running from two inches above his right ear downward then splitting into two fractures which extended approximately one inch below the ear.

"My examination showed the slightest distention just here," the colonel said, pointing to a spot on the plate. "Perhaps it is where he received a blow during the cave in. In any case, I think there is the appropriate site for a trepanation."

"Have you seen this type of injury before, doctor?"

"Not exactly the same, but similar. Relief of the cranial pressure provided improvement in each case. But you know each head injury can be very different. The brain is still very much an unknown. In one case, a young sergeant did well in the surgery but developed an infection and died three weeks later."

He was right, surgery is always a risk, but Ryan is not getting any better.

"I know what that is," Jonesy said.

Having just explained the surgery and need for it, I could see it had taken him by surprise.

"Will it stop this pain?"

"I think it will. We believe the pain is being caused by a buildup of pressure within your skull. The only way to relieve that pressure is through this surgery."

"When?"

"Right away. Sooner is better. I'll be in the operating theatre the entire time and during your recovery."

"And what of your leg?"

"If it remains clear, in another three or four days, Doctor Pinkerton will close the incision."

"Aren't we the pretty two," he said with a slight smile.

"I would say yes."

I turned to see Kathleen, in a robe and slippers. She looked pale, but steady.

She took a chair by the head of Jonesy's bed, putting her hand on top of his.

"I'm glad we are all together."

"Aye," Jonesy said. "A long way from the Somme."

"We have all seen too much of this war," I added.

"When will it end?" Kathleen asked.

"That is a question for the generals, my dear. But God, I hope it is soon."

I told Kathleen about the surgery before coming to see Jonesy.

"Ryan, I'll be back to duty within the week and will be able to help care for you during the recovery."

"That is the best news I've had in a long time."

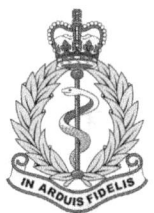

Chapter Thirty-Seven

"Now, I would have to let God take care of them."

General Hospital Number 14
Boulogne
5 August 1917

Ryan's surgery did not go well. He had a difficult time with the ether. The anesthesia produced nausea followed by vomiting. The fifteen minutes before he was under made me wonder if we could even proceed. Doctor Langdon did a marvelous job and had him stabilized and breathing normally for the operation.

The initial drilling with the trephine at the spot recommended by Doctor Pinkerton caused an additional fracture of the cranial structure. It is always a risk drilling in the vicinity of a fracture, but you can only make your best guess. He then used a Hudson hand brace to penetrate the material which had started to separate from the original fracture. Once under the second flap of bone, the epidural hematoma was visible. There was minimal bleeding, which told the doctor that the meningeal artery was not compromised. It raised my hopes that the damage would be minimal and relieving the pressure would solve the pain problem.

Doctor Pinkerton was then able to carefully remove the hematoma using a curette then suction. Saline irrigation was the used to clear any remaining blood. The concern was the amount of skull structure that was compromised. The doctor decided he would close the scalp for now. The dura was intact, which made Ryan a candidate for a cranial prosthesis. The current material used by the RAMC was aluminum, and it would be custom shaped and then attached in another surgery in several weeks.

I felt positive as I sat with Doctor Langdon waiting for Jonesy to come out of the anesthesia. He had as good a chance as anyone to live a normal life, barring any infection from this surgery or the next.

"You've known the corporal for some time?"

I laughed.

"We met the day a stepped off the ship in Le Havre. He was a motorcycle rider who then gave me a ride to the front in search of my battalion. He never left and immediately showed a remarkable affinity for the medical profession, becoming a medical orderly and my surgical assistant."

"Quite unusual, I would think."

"And we ended up doing unusual things for the last three years to take care of our lads. But I wouldn't have changed anything."

Thank God Jonesy's recovery from the ether went much more easily. With the oxygen to assist, he was back with us in short order. He was still going to be under the effects of morphine as we managed his post-operative pain. A difficult recovery, but I knew it was the only reasonable course of action. Now I would have to let God take care of him, with a little help from me.

For the next two days, Jonesy was very sedated with morphine injections every 4 hours. We used 10 mg due to his relatively light weight. Constant monitoring of his respiration and pulse was critical to ensure he did not succumb to respiratory distress.

I spent most of my waking hours next to his bed helping the nurses keep an eye on him. Those hours gave me a chance to consider what the two of us had been through since 1914. He had been with me every step of the way and never let me down or come up short. What more is there to say about a man? I found myself wanting to work with him after the war and hoped there was a way to make that happen. I know that he had no family to speak of, no connection to an area. Why not have him join me in Glasgow and assist in the practice? It would be a honorable career and always allow him to make a handsome way in the world. I think now is the time to propose my post war plans and see if he wanted to consider them a possibility.

My efforts continued for two full days. At that time, Doctor Pinkerton began to lower his dose of morphine and we watched as he rejoined the land of the living.

The afternoon of the third day after the operation, he was finally able to speak, although slowly and for only a short time. I went over the events of the surgery and his recovery, including the need for a follow up surgery to implant the prosthesis.

"Right," was his only response when I explained the need to put a metal plate in his head to replace the damaged bone. I knew that was the medication speaking and I would go into the process more in a couple of days.

He had not complained of head pain since coming out of the pain medication and I wondered if the pain was being masked by the morphine. Or, was the hematoma the only cause for the pain and now, he was truly on the road to recovery. If so, my prayers had been answered.

My leg continued to drain although it clearly was getting better. I felt I would be on time with a closure in the next several days. When I looked at the bandage, my thoughts always returned to those terrible moments in the trench. I truly did not regret what I had done and knew I was very lucky. The sheer arbitrariness of war had convinced me survival was just a matter of chance. The random artillery shell, a mine in the wrong place, a disease that you would never have encountered except for the horrific conditions of the battlefield. And yet when I go back to the battalion, I will not think of it. It always happens to someone else like James Edwards or Corey Timmons. At least that is what we all told ourselves.

Kathleen is now on light duty, which allows her to set her own hours and ease back into the rotation. It has been strange to be in a hospital bed knowing she is back at our cottage. The colonel expects I'll be on crutches for several days after the operation, but he will allow me to be an outpatient. If there are no complications, I will transition to a cane when able, then work to regain my strength. My intention is to return to the battalion in five or six weeks. The offensive is still going on and I know they will need all the medical support we can provide.

I'm hoping Jonesy's second surgery goes well and he can do his recovery here at the hospital. The idea of sending him into the massive military medical system is not something I want to consider. If he has a strong recovery, he could spend the rest of the war at the hospital as an orderly, out of harm's way and getting more experience in medicine.

I received a summons to Colonel Pinkerton's office three days after a successful operation to close my leg. Tired of wearing pajamas, I asked for help and was able to put on my uniform with one leg seam opened up to accommodate the bandage. The crutches were still my support for moving around and I felt very competent, even up and down stairs.

"Come in Doctor, and please sit down," I heard from the open door and entered with a smooth swing of the crutches. To my surprise, two men in uniform sat across from the colonel.

While not sure, I thought the uniforms were American, knowing that the yanks had been landing in France since the end of June.

"Gentlemen, this is Doctor David McFadden of the Highland Light Infantry. He's been in France since 1914 and seen every major battle to date. His bandage covers a bayonet wound suffered in a German trench as he was taking care of his wounded soldiers. I thought you would benefit from his experience which has included the actual battlefields along with the entire casualty evacuation system."

The two men looked at me as if I had three eyes but then both stood up and extended their hands.

"Doctor, I am Tom Fairburn, I'll be the main A.E.F liaison officer with your medical staff." His handshake was firm and his manner very collegial.

The second man, who was a bit older, said, "Lawrence Dye, I'll be the senior surgeon in this area of the front for our troops."

So, the Americans were finally here. After years of wondering what they would do and hoping they would join the effort to defeat Germany it was really going to happen. I just wondered how long it would take for them to really have any serious effect on the battlefield.

We spent the next three hours, including lunch, discussing a myriad of subjects. By the end of our time together I was actually worn down, but glad I could help them get one step in front of all of the problems we had encountered over the last three years.

I was using a cane when Jonesy underwent his prothesis operation. The procedure went well, and he was able to finally see the light at the end of the tunnel. His attitude was good and he realized staying at the hospital would be the best thing for him. Doctor Pinkerton was very amenable to my proposal, and I knew Jonesy would do well in Pinkerton's hospital.

After the operation, the next two weeks were truly a blessing. I was not physically ready to return to the battalion. My task was to continue my recovery in preparation for full duty. But in my mind, my job was to enjoy the time with my wife and forget about the front.

To that end, my time in Boulogne was wonderful. I think both our experiences with sickness and injury gave us a deep appreciation for what we had and were able to enjoy. Despite the relatively short time we had lived together as man and wife, our newly renewed closeness had a different feel about it. The whirlwind of our wedding and return to France never gave us the chance to relax and enjoy the pleasure of each other's company. Now we had time to talk, hold each other and revel in the day to day events of a life together.

The time went all too fast.

While only fifty miles from Boulogne to Poperinge, it took my car and driver almost six hours to negotiate the muddy roads, stalled convoys and the occasional German aircraft looking for targets.

Using my cane as minimally as possible, I found the battalion commander in his admin tent.

"Reporting, sir."

"Doctor, it is good to see you."

We shook hand and he motioned me to a camp chair.

"How's your leg?"

"A little stiff, but getting better every day."

"I received notification yesterday that you have been awarded a bar to your Distinguished Service Cross for your defense of the wounded during the German counter-attack."

My mind returned to that moment in the trench. The DSC was for bravery, not what I had done.

"Colonel, I was simply trying to stay alive, there was no bravery involved."

He looked at me and shook his head.

"David, you showed bravery by even being in the trench. You told Corporal Chesney you would station yourself outside the dugout to deal with the Germans. That takes a great deal of bravery. And you ended up in hand-to-hand combat, which prevented any harm coming to the men in the dugout."

"Yes, sir," I said, just let it be.

"Doctors Rossi and Bernard have done a superb job filling in for you. I think one or both deserve some leave now that we are looking at two to three weeks here in the rear area."

"Is the offensive over?"

"It has failed, but headquarters continues to throw men at the ridges around Passchendaele. Barring a major German push, which I very much doubt, the campaign of 1917 is drawing to a close. The great question is when and how the Americans will go into action. So far, their numbers are not overwhelming and many of their troops still need additional training. My guess is a major combined offensive in the spring. That would give the Americans time to get more troops in place and trained. The French have a new commander, Petain, but he has his hands full right now with mutinies and a demoralized army. He'll need time to get ready to fight."

"So, we lick our wounds, rebuild the battalion and hope for a quiet fall."

"That is the plan, David. Now we just need to have it unfold that way."

I found Glen Rossi in a tent which had a simple sign outside, "Medical."

His eyes immediately went to my leg and cane as he stood and offered his hand.

"Ah, the world is back in line, McFadden has returned."

"And how is Canada's favorite son?"

He smiled.

"Damn glad that we have been pulled out of that slaughter house."

"What was the butcher's bill?"

"During the last two weeks on the line, we lost thirty-seven killed and sixty wounded."

"And what progress?"

"We now own some mud that used to be German mud. I'm sure that General Haig has been given another medal."

I didn't blame him for his anger. The cost of men with no measurable gain has been the story of the Western Front. Hundreds of thousands of men killed and crippled for nothing. Now I was getting angry.

"How's Jonesy?"

"He was doing well when I left. The placement of the plate went well, and I think he will make a full recovery."

"Thank God for that."

"Doctor Pinkerton plans to keep him at the hospital and let him take over orderly duties. I don't want him shipped home and he sure as hell can't come back here."

Glen looked at my leg.

"You don't look very spry if you ask me, doctor."

"Stiff and sore, but it's getting better."

"Right."

"Really, it is."

"Damned English, you can lie with such conviction."

Damned Canadian could see right through me.

Over the next several days, I was able to catch up with Glenn and Rand. Both bore the signs of too much time taking care of wounded young men. I encouraged both of them to take leave. Rand jumped on the chance to return to England and see his fiance. Glenn told me he just needed to sleep a great deal and drink some good whiskey.

Jimmy Chesney, was now wearing the stripes of a sergeant and leading the medical staff, which consisted of himself, Private Sutton, Private Barnsby and Corporal Dwyer. Barnsby and Dwyer had arrived during my time in hospital. The younger Barnsby was fresh out of training, while Dwyer had been working casualty clearing stations for the last two years. According to Glenn Rossi, both seemed competent and were fitting in well.

"Those stripes look very good on you, sergeant."

Jimmy grinned at me.

"Doctor, it is good to see you. Almost good as new?

We shook hands.

"Jimmy, I don't have to be good as new, I have you."

He looked serious.

"I will do my best, sir."

I slapped him on the back.

"You always have. For three years I have seen you take on every challenge and come out on top. We are a great team and the battalion knows it. Now, tell me about the new lads."

A week later, Glen found me in my tent. He had what looked like official correspondence in his hand.

"David, you will be happy to know that the RAMC in all their wisdom has decided that surgical capability must be closer to the front. In fact, Advanced Dressing Stations would be put in place at Casualty Clearing Stations. They would have portable x-ray stations and be equipped to conduct surgical operations, particularly on time sensitive abdominal and cranial injuries."

"I'll be damned. It only took them three years."

"Oh, it doesn't end. Thomas splints will be available at all unit levels and directed for use on all femur fractures."

"Will wonders never cease?"

"And it goes on to say that Carrel-Dakin continuous irrigation and regular times dressing changes will now be standard operating procedure. They are even formalizing triage procedures for use at the clearing stations."

It was known that change always comes slowly in the military, until the situation becomes critical. At least we have won some of the medical battles, perhaps next time it won't take so long.

We made one more move up to the front lines in 1917. Once in position, the only action the battalion saw was patrols and trench raids. But men still get wounded and killed on patrols. Now the weather began to attack our lads as well. Influenza, trench foot and dysentery began to cut through the battalion as they had last winter. But the British Tommy did what he always has done, soldier on no matter what. At least this year, the winter clothes were issued in time, and we didn't have to rely on donations from home to survive the cold.

Perhaps it was the weather, or the time of year, but it felt very much like we were the forgotten army. While we had been here for over three years, the Americans seemed to be all anyone could talk about. At the same time, events in Russia were leading to talk that the Russians would drop out of the war. It was a very unsettled time.

In November we received word that a revolution had taken place in Russia, with the Bolsheviks taking control of many cities. The army apparently had been deserting the battlefield since the summer, and the Germans now had no enemy facing them in the east. The question was when those German soldiers would move to the west and go into action against us. While the Americans would be adding their numbers to ours, the German armies coming from the Russian Front were experienced combat troops. The Americans had seen no real action since arriving in France. The future seemed dark, and we all wondered if we were going to endure another year of war.

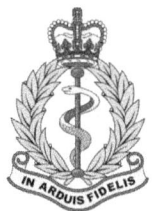

Chapter Thirty-Eight

"I wanna go back, me mates are the best."

General Hospital Number 14
Boulogne
2 December 1917

Once on the road back to the front, the evidence of the Americans was clear. Convoys heading east with loaded trucks, towed artillery pieces and mounted cavalry. A new army of men that would hopefully turn the tide against Germany. It seemed England had been bled dry over the last three years. We needed fresh troops, supplies and spirit if there was any chance of breaking the stalemate on the front.

With the battalion settled into winter quarters and the level of activity at the front low, I took the opportunity to make the trip to Boulogne to see Kathleen and Jonesy. Her letters kept me up on the latest from the hospital and I was looking forward to time with her. She let me know Jonesy was well employed and had made a great impression on the doctors and nurses alike. While still only twenty-one years of age, his maturity from three years at war gave him a strong sense of purpose as he went about his duties. In a surprise to me, she had begun assisting in surgery again in addition to her ward duties.

On arrival I went directly to Doctor Pinkerton's office, hoping to catch him and pay my respects.

"David, please come in. And I see no cane."

"No sir, still a little stiffness, but other than that, your surgical ability left me with a perfectly serviceable leg."

"That is wonderful! What brings you here, other than a desire to see your lovely wife?"

"I will admit that is my main motive, but I also wanted to check on my old orderly, Corporal Jones."

"Jonesy, of course. He has settled in quite well and I think has truly helped the nurses deal with the toughest cases. Having spent so much time on the line, he can explain things to then that make their care better."

"For a young man, he has always impressed me with his ability and desire."

"Would that all orderlies were cut from the same cloth."

An idea crossed my mind.

"Doctor, for a good deal of time, he assisted me in surgery. He was very good and I think he actually has future in medicine after the war. Perhaps you might use him in the same manner."

The colonel nodded as he considered my idea.

"Let me think about that. There might well be a way to develop him into a true surgical assistant. It has always been the domain of the nurse, but why not utilize motivated young men?"

I found Jonesy in Ward Three talking with a young soldier with both legs heavily bandaged. The two seemed to be enjoying their conversation, the wounded soldier gesturing with both hands. Standing behind Jonesy, I heard them talking about what the next step would be for the young man. He looked up at me and Jonesy turned, grinned and stood up.

We shook hands and told each other hello.

"Who is your patient here, Ryan?"

"Private Booth, sir, from the West Lancashires."

He looked to be barely of age, maybe eighteen, but likely younger. I picked up the chart and saw he had multiple shrapnel injuries to both legs. Nothing immediately life threatening, but a long and painful surgery to remove the metal from his legs.

"What happened, Private Booth?"

"One of them minewerfer things."

"Indeed," I said, "Nasty wounds, I'm afraid. But something we can take good care of in no time."

He smiled.

"I wanna go back, me mates are the best."

The enthusiasm of youth. But after being wounded, not all soldiers want to return to the fight.

"Do what the doctors and nurses tell you and you'll be out of here in no time."

"Corporal, do you have a minute?"

Over a cup of tea in the dining area, we were able to relax and catch up. I told him of the changes at the battalion, and he related his recovery and going back on duty.

"Sometimes, I do get a headache, but they don't last long, and I just need aspirin to get by. And, I haven't had one in some time, so maybe they're going away."

"That's good, but any time you have a bad headache, you let the doctors know."

"Aye, I know I have a metal plate in my head, so I have to be careful."

"I talked to Colonel Pinkerton about you becoming a surgical assistant."

He was silent for a moment, then said, "I would like to do that."

"With your experience and how you like to learn about medicine, it would be a perfect spot for you to take the next step."

"The next step?"

"Certainly. You could be my surgical assistant in my new medical practice when the war is over."

He turned to look at me.

"Are you serious?"

"Of course, I am. I'll be a surgeon, and I need an assistant to help me in the operating room. I've been thinking about it and I may specialize in helping wounded and disfigured soldiers get better."

He smiled.

"I'll learn everything I can here, I promise."

"Ryan, there is no doubt in my mind about that."

"This reminds me of the fishing lodge on Barr Loch," I said, looking at the beams on the ceiling of our bedroom in the cottage.

Kathleen rolled over and looked at me with a smile.

"I suppose both places will have good memories, if you know what I mean."

Her playful nature was never evident in public, but my wife was a delight to be around. My leave had been a wonderful interlude in the day-to-day grind of the war. We enjoyed Jeanne's cooking, wonderful wine and the ability to walk together in the crisp winter days.

The occasional storm reminded me that with the spring would come another year of battle. Unless the governments came to some agreement. My expectations of that were nil, it seemed that only a military victory would finally end this terrible war. The Germans would be reinforced by their troops returning from the east, while the Americans would fill out our armies. It seemed to me all that was going to happen was an even greater loss of life and with the two sides in a perennial stalemate, nothing would really change. The thought was depressing, but the thought that I have kept with me is what my father told me in 1914, "do your duty." That is all I can do.

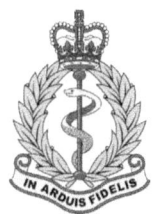

Chapter Thirty-Nine

"Right now we were spread too thin."

Highland Light Infantry
Near St Quentin
18 March 1918

Once on the road back to the front, the evidence of the Americans was clear. Convoys heading east with loaded trucks, towed artillery pieces and mounted cavalry. A new army of men that would hopefully turn the tide against Germany. It seemed England had been bled dry over the last three years. We needed fresh troops, supplies and spirit if there was any chance of breaking the stalemate on the front.

Everyone knew the Germans were preparing for a spring offensive, but where they would attack was the question. Bits and pieces of rumor, intelligence and sparse reports let those of us in the field know that there had been a large buildup of supplies, including rail lines in the area of the Somme sector. We knew the uncomfortable truth that the British Fifth Army was spread very thin in the area. The army had seen the final result of the massive loss of men in 1917 and a number of battalions were disbanded due to a lack of personnel. While conscription was pulling more men into active service, they were not in the field yet ready for combat. It begged the question, could we mount an offensive that cost us the massive losses we saw in 1916 and 1917? There must be a critical level of troops needed to continue fighting. We could only hope the Americans would be ready when the Germans attacked and that our replacements would arrive soon. Right now, we were simply spread too thin.

"Good morning, sergeant."

"Top of the morning, captain. There's coffee on the stove."

As always, Sergeant Bill Nance had the department ready for another day of training and equipment distribution. We continued our policy that each bearer would carry a medical bag and also undergo as much training as time allowed. Rand Bernard and Glen Rossi were ready to man the aid stations, while myself and Dan Jennings had the surgery ready for action.

I helped myself to the coffee, which was hot and most welcome.

"Sergeant, the colonel has called an officer's call at nine. I don't think it will be more than an hour. If you get the training started, I'll join when I'm done with the colonel."

Our training this morning would focus on the bearers. I was comfortable that our old hands were ready, but the new crews needed all of the indoctrination we could provide. I knew it would save lives if we trained them well.

"Gentlemen, I have the latest intelligence summary from Division. This is current as of late last evening."

Colonel Prescott stood in front of the battalion officers, some of which were taking notes.

"Aerial reconnaissance flights have confirmed more troop buildups in the area between the Somme and St Quentin. The recent arrival of additional artillery units leads the staff to believe an attack, when it comes, will likely be aimed at this section of the line. Captured prisoners have noted stormtrooper units are in place among the regular infantry units. A logical objective for any attack would be Amiens, which is key to our logistic support for this entire sector. It goes without saying that taking Amiens would the pose a critical threat to Paris."

A question from the audience asked, "Who will we be facing?"

"We think the German Second Army. They are under the overall command of the Crown Prince of Bavaria. Our intelligence people consider the Second Army experienced and effective. We also know that the sign of an attack are clear, it could come at any time. We will fully man our trenches and dugout commencing today. I would like a report from each company commander when his men are deployed.

I suspected everyone was thinking what I was, this will be a nasty fight. It seems like the final rounds in a prize fight, each combatant will try to throw their hardest punch. But I knew we were understrength and many of our new men had never seen combat other than patrols.

Walking back to the medical admin tent with Glen and Rand we didn't talk much. What was there to say? Our men were as trained as we could get them. They all had their necessary equipment and were ready for whatever the Germans might throw at them. The big question now was when the enemy would attack.

"We'll need to man the aid stations now to be ready. I think it will be just like the lads in the trenches. Take your blankets and plan on sleeping there. We'll stay in contact, and I'll make sure your rations are delivered."

"Would that include any libations?" Glen asked.

I could only smile.

"Most certainly, I do know you are Canadian and have your needs."

This area of the front was well supplied with rear area dugouts which were suited well for the forward aid stations. Glen and Rand picked out sites behind our main trench, but accessible by communication trenches and ravines. But as we learned with James, dugouts will not protect from direct artillery hits. I remembered the briefing from the colonel talking about additional artillery being spotted behind the German lines. Their artillery had always been deadly, but more could only be worse.

Back at the surgical dugout, we got busy adding some more protection for the operating area. The Royal Engineers provided empty bags for filling and the sergeant major detailed a squad to help us build protective walls around the open part of the access. While nothing could protect from a direct hit, these bags could do a good job against the flying debris and shrapnel. A strange way to practice medicine.

Dan sat on a camp chair, his tunic off and his undershirt sweat soaked after hours filling the bags. There was no one near him, but he normally was alone. I think the damage to his ability to speak had led him to turn inward. But you always sensed a man who was communicating with you whether he was talking or not. It seemed he was always the first one to pitch in when something needed to be done. What would he have done without the big man, I don't know.

I pulled up a chair and sat down next to him.

"Thank you," I said.

He turned to look at me.

"For what," he rasped.

"For everything you have done so well for this battalion and me."

A slight smile appeared on his lips and he nodded.

I nodded back. A truly good man.

I felt the surgery was in good shape. For the first time it seemed the medical supplies were in good supply. The army finally solved the supply problem just as the recruiting and training programs had fallen short. The sergeant major told me the battalion was one hundred and fifty soldiers short of full manning. I wasn't sure how that would affect the battle, but it had to have some effect. Many of the troopers had not seen action and it was always a shock the first time. I remember the colonel talking about the stormtrooper units. The soldiers I encountered when I was bayoneted were from one of the stormtrooper units. They were fierce fighters, and I hope our lads didn't have to deal with any more of them. Only time would tell.

Two days of continued preparations began to lull us into a sense that this attack was not going to happen. On the morning of the 23rd, we found out how wrong we were.

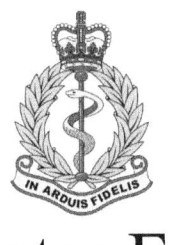

Chapter Forty

"Dan, they're taking you to a hospital."

Highland Light Infantry
Near St Quentin
23 March 1918

We were awakened in the early hours of the morning to the explosions of an artillery barrage. The tempo of explosions told me this was a major effort by the Germans as shells burst every two seconds up and down the front. In a moment it seemed as if we had been swallowed by a beast, with every sense assaulted. The barrage lasted for two hours. It was difficult to imagine the number of artillery rounds the Germans were expending on this attack.

After two hours, it was clear to me this was going to be the major attack we had been awaiting. At least the battalion was already in place, under cover and ready to repulse the Germans. When I climbed out of the dugout to take in the surrounding area, I could see little left intact through the mist and smoke. Any structure in the area, tent, building or supply dump was destroyed. I realized we were lucky to still be alive.

Dan and I had sat in the dugout for the entire attack. As we learned so many years ago, in an artillery barrage, you just take cover and let the barrage expend itself. There was nowhere to run and any attempt was likely to result in an unfavorable result.

The sound of machine gun fire told me something was happening at the main trench. Was this the German attack beginning? How bad had our men be hurt in the shelling? While no patients had arrived, I didn't expect any during the shelling. The area between the main trench and our dugout was wide open and any attempt by the stretcher bearers to make that trip would have been foolish. Now that the bombardment had stopped, we could expect the flow of casualties to begin.

Our first arrival was not a casualty, but Sergeant Nance. He entered the dugout, smelling of cordite and dust.

"Doctor, the German attack is rolling our lines back."

"What does that mean?"

"Some of our men have had to fall back to the reserve trench and set up holding points."

"What now?"

He shook his head.

"I'm not sure we can hold the main line. If the battalion falls back, your position here is going to be right in the middle of the battle."

This had never happened before, and I had not thought about falling back. Where to go and what to take? The ambulances were still at the CCS. We have no way to move our supplies.

"What do you suggest?"

Nance wiped the sweat off his face.

"Get moving now, take whatever we can carry and find a place to set up an aid station. I expect our other two aid stations will be doing the same."

Without a truck or wagon, we could only carry medical bags and the most basic of supplies. There were bags already packed for the bearers, and we could take those. I would take my general medical bag. But how far do we go, or where?

"All right, let's get our bags together and we'll leave now."

Dan nodded and picked up two bags, heading up the ramp out of the dugout.

Suddenly the staccato sound of machine gun fire echoed in the dugout, followed by the sound of an engine. I hesitated for a moment, then went up the ramp, just as another fusillade of fire echoed off the walls, the second engine sound made me look up and I saw a German airplane flash past at a very low altitude.

Dan lay on his side, one of the medical bags torn open, bandages laying open on the ground.

The amount blood told me this was a potentially fatal wound. His leg below the knee was horribly damaged with white bone visible through torn flesh and much blood.

I found a webbing strap tourniquet in the medical bag and cut open Dan's trouser to get at his thigh. Attaching the web, I tightened it as quickly as I could to stop the flow of blood.

Dan was making a moaning sound, rocking slightly, his face contorted in pain.

"Dan, hold on. Let me get this on and I'll get the morphine."

Bill Nance slipped down next to me, a morphine syringe ready for injection.

"Morphine?" he asked.

"Go ahead."

He injected the medicine under the skin on Dan's exposed thigh. I knew this was risky, but his pain justified the chance the morphine might lower his blood pressure. It was a tradeoff I had to take.

The sound of machine gun and rifle fire was getting louder.

"We need to move," Nance said.

Looking around, I saw a stretcher on the ground.

"Get him on that," I said.

We carefully rolled Dan on the stretcher, and I covered his leg with an open bandage to cover the wound. The damage was extensive, and I knew that amputation was the likely outcome.

With my medical bag, pistol and two canteens, I picked up the stretcher with the sergeant. It was now up to us to get Dan to safety.

Pressing two men we found in a dugout into service, the four of us carried Dan toward the rear area. He was no longer moaning, the morphine having taken effect.

The effects of the German artillery continued as we moved west. The few structures along our course of march were damaged or destroyed. A small farmhouse was just a shell of a building. If we could find some reasonable shelter, I wanted to examine Dan and set up an aid station.

Our search was rewarded when we found a deep crater, with the remains of a trench and dugout still visible. There were plenty of sandbags laying across the crater and the remains of the timber that had reinforced the trench. I estimated we were two miles from our original surgery site.

Soldiers pulling back became more obvious, not just single men, but several together moving as you would expect a squad might. Was the battalion setting up a defensive position here? If so, we might want to move further back to stay out of the line of fire.

As I examined Dan's lower leg, I knew only one course of action made sense. The leg must be amputated. Three inches below the knee would clear the shattered bone and leave him a knee joint. But we needed to get him to a casualty clearing station.

"We need an ambulance or some vehicle to get him to the CCS."

Nance nodded.

We could hear more activity over the ridge of the crater, which told me the battalion was falling back. Would this turn into a breach of the line, or could the lads set up a viable defense?

"Give me twenty minutes. I'll see what might still be in the area. Maybe some of the drivers panicked and left their trucks."

Only if there is a God in heaven, I thought.

The intensity of rifle fire increased after the sergeant left. Several soldiers climbed over the edge of the crater and set up firing positions.

"Let anyone know, this is an aid station," I yelled at the men. Two heard me and waved an acknowledgment. While I didn't have much in the way of supplies, I could take care of soldiers wounds using their own field dressing packets.

More men joined us in the crater and I recognized Herb Turley as he slid down below the rim. I watched him reload his pistol and then he saw me.

"What's happening," I yelled over the rifle fire.

He crawled over to me.

"The battalion is pulling back. We'll try to delay the Germans and eventually stop them, but right now, we just have to save the battalion."

"Have you seen Prescott?"

If the battalion was to survive, the commander was the key.

"My last order came by runner, but he was alive thirty minutes ago."

"Can I do anything," I asked.

"Stay alive," he said then turned to his men setting up a machine gun.

Looking around, it was clear to me that moving was out of the question. I would stay here, tend the wounded and hope Bill Nance finds some help.

I took the chance to re-examine Dan's leg. Thank God his blood loss was now minimal and I loosened the tourniquet briefly. It took only a moment for me to tighten it back. He was going to lose the leg and keeping blood loss to a minimum was critical.

Two soldiers came over the edge of the crater, a wounded man supported between them.

"Over here," I yelled.

They lay the man on the ground and fell on their knees, clearly exhausted.

"He's hit in the back," one man said.

"Help me roll him over."

The man's tunic showed no sign of a wound on his frontal torso as we turned him on his back. The blood from a wound was evident, but he was not bleeding excessively.

"What's your name, soldier?"

"Adams, Sammy Adams," the man said the pain clear in his strained voice.

"All right, Sammy, rest easy."

The wound appeared to a tear, perhaps by a bullet tumbling. The impact was in the infrascapular region three inches from mid-line. My initial concern was damage to the lungs and or heart, but he was having no problem breathing. This could be a spent bullet deflected off a rib. I think a dressing and morphine will take care of Sammy Adams for now.

With my first patient bandaged and resting, I moved sandbags to provide more protection for the soldier.

There were now over thirty men in the crater and I watched Herb deploy them along the rim. Another group of five men appeared at the edge, carrying a Lewis machine gun. The very distinctive barrel and ammunition pan magazine was a comforting sight. Resting on a tripod, it gave our men a very effective weapon if the Germans tried to storm our position. The other men were carrying extra ammunition for the gun, which also provided more confidence in our defense. The gun crew began to place the gun in position, using some of the sandbags and timber for protection.

I watched as the young men prepared themselves for the German attack. I saw two men sharing ammunition, several others lighting cigarettes. Herb sent two men to look for ammunition and the gun crew fired a short burst. Now we wait.

The sound of men sliding into crater behind me was the arrival of the battalion commander and three other soldiers.

"Hello doctor," the colonel said, in a very conversational tone.

"Good morning, colonel."

Before I could add anything, he turned to Herb Turley and they were calmly discussing the current situation. Their experience was obvious as was their professional demeanor. Was that natural or an effort on their part? But I knew each man and they were steady as the day is long. I was proud to be part of their battalion.

"I'll be moving on down the line, doctor. Is there anything I can do for you?"

"All set here, we'll take good care of the lads."

"Right. Thank you."

The four men scrambled over the top of the crater and were gone.

The attack came two hours after the visit by Colonel Prescott. Thankfully, the respite had given the battalion time to establish a defensive line and resupply the men with ammunition and water.

Sergeant Nance returned with four men to carry Dan to an evacuation point where there were vehicles to take him to a casualty clearing station.

"Dan, they're taking you to a hospital," I told him, not sure if he would understand through the morphine.

He opened his eyes, which told me he was aware of what I said.

"Make sure he gets to the CCS," I said as the soldiers picked up the stretcher.

"You want me to go with him?" Nance asked.

I nodded.

Was I losing my objectivity? Probably, I told myself, but the survival of that man was important to me, and I think I have earned the right to be a little selfish.

The German troops kept up their attack for just over an hour. The battalion held the line and eventually the enemy pulled back out of range of our guns. Several of the men were wounded and one was killed when he was hit in the face with a bullet.

We were surprised when the order came down the line to fall back at 8:00 PM. A small rear guard would remain to make the line appear fully manned while the majority of the battalion would fall back two miles to fill in a solid defense line that was being put in place. I was thankful it would give me a chance to rebuild my aid station and find out what had happened to Glen and Rand during the German assault.

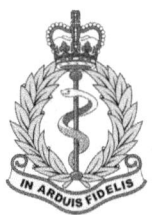

Chapter Forty-One

"... I wondered if this could possibly be the end of this nightmare."

Highland Light Infantry
Just east of Amiens
22 April 1918

For two weeks, the battalion fought a desperate battle with the German assault troops. The slaughter of men on both sides rivalled anything seen at the Battle of the Somme or Passchendaele. By the time of their farthest advance, which turned out to be April 5th, the battalion had lost fifty percent of our men, killed or wounded. The failure of the enemy to advance any further led us to believe they had run out of reserves. Reports from up and down the line reflected what we were seeing, German units dug in, but receiving no support from their rear.

We were receiving supplies, but no replacement soldiers. Some Americans were arriving to support us, and the assistance was gratefully accepted. I saw a number of medical personnel in and around the casualty control station and at the front.

Our little band survived with the wounding of Dan Jenning being our only casualty. My prayer of thanks was heartfelt, and I knew we had been fortunate.

This latest phase of the war seemed like a prize fight. One fighter came out punching until he was worn out. The other fended off the blows but survive the onslaught. Now we were in between rounds. What would happen now?

Colonel Prescott was called away to several meetings and the impression we all had was that the allies, now reinforced by the Americans, would launch our own offensive. For the Highland Light Infantry, we needed men and time to integrate them into the battalion. If we were lucky, the offensive would not start for several months, but as we had learned so well, logic does not always drive events.

I looked at my watch, seeing there was twenty minutes before the battalion officer's call. The lack of any significant activity on the front lines over the last two weeks had sparked speculation that the Germans were pulling back. My experience told me the Germans seldom withdrew without being forced back. Perhaps the colonel had new intelligence.

"Time for a cup of coffee?"

Corporal Dwyer was carrying a large pitcher, the steam coming out of the pour spout.

"Fresh from the cook tent?"

"Yes, sir."

"I would enjoy a cup, I have ten minutes before I have to go and hot coffee might help take the chill off."

Our medical tent was located only five minutes from the commander's gathering point he used for our daily briefings.

As I sat down to enjoy my coffee, Glen Rossi came around the corner of the tent, carrying an open piece of paper.

"Good morning, Lieutenant Rossi, how are you today?"

"Wishing I was back in Vancouver, if truth be known," he snapped back, a grin on his face. He held out the paper to me.

"What's this?"

"Read it, it's good news."

I looked down at the letter which had been opened already.

It was from Colonel Pinkerton, and my eyes quickly scanned the page, afraid it might be bad news about Kathleen. But it was about Dan Jennings. He was recovering following the amputation and to this point there had been no complications. Thank the Lord. The colonel felt he would be ready to transport back to England within three to four weeks, depending on how the stump healed. My only thought was I needed to see him before he was evacuated. There would be a happy ending to this if I had anything to say about it.

"Wonderful news," I said to Glen.

"Truly it is."

"I'll try to see him before he leaves for England."

"He'll appreciate that."

"I'm going to offer him a job."

Rossi turned to me.

"What did you say?"

"I want to make him part of my practice after the war."

The Canadian looked at me askance.

"You're serious?"

"Indeed, but now I have the colonel's meeting. Back in an hour I expect."

There were a number of new faces at the meeting. Most were young and obviously the replacements for the battalion officers who were killed or wounded in the last month.

Prescott was already there, sitting on a sandbag wall reading from a folder. He looked at his watch and stood up turning to look over the group.

"Good morning, gentlemen. I have received some most interesting intelligence. Here are two excerpts from letter intercepted on their was from the army back to Germany.

"The men are exhausted. They believed the offensive would bring peace. But all they see are our soldiers left behind in the mud. How many more will die in this useless war?"

"We are understrength, short of food and ammunition. The enemy seems to always have more troops and we get no replacements. What do the generals think they can do?"

He looked up from the folder, "There are reports of strikes in Berlin and other major cities demanding food and an end to the war. It is clear this is the time for a major push by the allied armies. The Americans will soon have well over a million fresh troops ready to go into battle. With our increase in aircraft and the new iron monsters, we have a tactical advantage. Now is the time to finish this war."

As I walked back to our area I wondered if this could possibly be the end of this nightmare. I would pray the colonel was right.

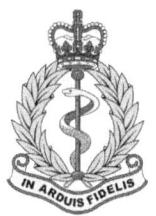

Chapter Forty-Two

"He's paid a price and that's no error."

General Hospital Number 14
Boulogne
6 May 1918

One week of leave came as the battalion was pulled back to one of the rear area training camps. Now at three quarters strength, it was time to indoctrinate the new arrivals. Glen and Rand would conduct exams of the new arrivals and I did not have to be present for that evolution. A chance to see Kathleen and Jonesy was precious, to be able to talk with Dan Jennings, critical. I knew that the loss of his leg would be a severe blow. Before the war, he was a postal worker. A wound like this would prevent him from returning to the mail service and cast a pall over his future. But I had a plan.

My first task was to find Kathleen. The matron at the front desk told me she was on her rotation to surgery, which she did along with her duties on Ward D. Unfortunately, she was in the operating theatre and there was no way to know when she might be free. Doctor Pinkerton was also in surgery, so my attempt at paying my respects would have to wait.

Walking across the yard to the casino brought back memories of my time at the hospital. Doing what I always thought I wanted to do, each day, one surgery after another. But now I don't think I see myself at one of the big London hospitals, part of the very structured organization, run by the senior surgeons. I saw that during my training and know full well what it is like.

Sitting down on one of the benches near the casino entrance I let my imagination run. Why not take my experience back to Glasgow? Open my own practice or join my father's. I wanted to know my patients and take care of them like I had done in the battalion. Why not build my own team with Jonesy, and Kathleen. Glen Rossi might even want to be part of it. And there would be a position for Dan. One leg or two, he had so much to offer to a team or the patients of that team. Suddenly the dark years of the war were giving way to a bright future for all of us.

Katheen was taking off her mask as she came around a corner from the operating room. Her hair was covered with a scarf and the mask coming off reminded me how utterly beautiful she was.

"Kathleen!"

She turned toward me, the mask in one hand.

"David!"

The two of us were oblivious to the other members of the surgical team in the corridor, who walked by quietly, respecting our privacy.

My arms around Kathleen, I moved us to the side of the hall as the patient on a gurney came out of the operating room.

"What a nice way to end a surgical session," Doctor Pinkerton said, pulling off his gloves and removing his mask.

I extended my hand, which the colonel firmly grasped.

"It is good to see you, David. Stop by when you get settled," he said, nodding to Kathleen. "If your wife will let you go for a few minutes."

He smiled and continued down the corridor.

Turning back to Kathleen, I kissed her on the lips and reveled to be with my wife again.

Walking back to the hospital, Kathleen asked, "How long can you stay?"

"A week, but the battalion has pulled back to the Abbeville Training Area. I think we'll be there for some time, so I think I'll be able to get more leave in a couple of weeks."

"I hope so," she said, squeezing my arm. "Have you seen Ryan?"

"No, I wanted to see you first."

"And I would expect nothing else. But he will be so happy to see you."

"Have you seen Dan Jennings?"

"Every day. He's doing as well as could be expected with a terrible wound like that."

"I need to see him."

"He will like that, I am sure."

"He needs to look to the future and I'm going to give him a reason."

She turned to look at me.

"That sounds quite interesting and a bit mysterious."

"I will invite him to become a member of my new medical practice I will open in Glasgow."

"Oh my, that was unexpected."

"Kathleen, this war has changed me. I think I know what I want to do in medicine, and I can do that in Glasgow, far from the pomp of London."

"I hope I'm included in your plan," she said with a hint of sarcasm.

"You, my dear will be our chief surgical assistant, working alongside our medical assistant, Ryan Jones. Our office supervisor will be one Daniel Jennings, late of the British army."

"My, you have been busy."

"It will be wonderful, we can run our practice the way a medical operation should be run. We'll look at our patients as people and take care of them as individuals. And for those who are of lesser means, we will be understanding."

Kathleen stopped and took my arm. She raised her face to mine and kissed me on the lips.

"I like your plan, doctor."

I literally ran into Jonesy, coming around a corner on the second floor by C Ward.

"Strike me pink," he exclaimed as we separated ourselves.

"I was looking for you, and now I have most certainly have found you."

We clasped each other's hand.

"You're looking well," he said. "No ill effects from the last run in with Jerry?

"We were all lucky, no one was hurt except Dan."

Jonesy's face turned serious.

"He's getting along, but it's been tough."

"How so?"

"I think the leg was the topping to the voice and his eye. He's paid a price and that's no error."

"Let's go see him"

C Ward was almost full, and Jonesy led me to the far end of the first row of beds. I could see the big man in the last bed, under a window.

His eyes were closed as we walked up, but they opened as we reached the bedside.

"Hello, Dan," I said.

"Good…to see you," he said quietly, the rasp barely audible.

"Took me longer to get up here than I wanted, but I had to come and see you."

"You...Nance saved my life."

"And I'm damned glad we were able to. But it took a tough man to hang on through the last attack."

His eyes showed he was remembering something no one would want to recall.

"And you'll recover and get on with life, which is what all of us have to do after the last four years."

I looked at Ryan, and said, "The three of us have been here for the whole thing. Now it's time for all of us to think about the future."

"Hard to do," Dan said.

"You worked for the Post Office before the war, right?"

He nodded.

"Do you want to go back to it?"

"Hard to deliver the post."

"Ah, yes."

"How would you like to work for me?" I asked.

His eyes opened wider.

"You?"

"I'll have my own medical practice in Glasgow. Ryan and my wife will assist me in surgery, but I need someone as the office supervisor."

"Super?"

"That's right. Taking care of all the things to run the practice. Scheduling patients, ordering supplies, taking care of billing and you'll have a clerk or two working for you."

For a moment I thought he didn't hear me, then he smiled the sheepish smile we all knew.

"Very good."

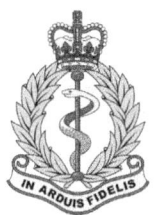

Chapter Forty-Three

"... there will be a great effort to not be the last man killed in this war."

Highland Light Infantry
Mons, Belgium
7 November 1918

The cold at the front was something I never got used to. This fall had been no different. Despite the intensity of the fighting and speed of advance, when the winds blew and the rain poured, noting else seemed important. The fighting had been intense, as the combined allied armies forced the German army back toward Germany. The years of static warfare in the world of trenches were forgotten as the enemy army was pushed hard back from their prepared positions.

The battalion never was brought back up to full strength, the manpower pool having been drained by four years of slaughter. But the troops were experienced and given a chance to fight in the open fields were magnificent. It was as if the pent up frustration of trench warfare had been thrown aside and our lads attacked with a renewed energy. The result was a series of victories over the demoralized Germans. Over the last six weeks, both in the Battles of Selle and Sambre, the near final blows were delivered. Now the question was how the final coup de grace would be administered.

"Perhaps they are dragging the war out so we will get to spend one more Christmas in the frozen fields of France or Germany, what say you?"

Glen Rossi had a woolen cap pulled down over his ears and a scarf wrapped tightly around his throat. He sat down, rubbing his hands together.

"It is a plot by the high command, certainly."

"Blast his cold, my hands are done for."

"Where are your gloves," I asked.

"Lost them," he said, clenching his hands into fists and blowing on them."

I laughed.

"Here, the coffee's hot, it'll warm you."

He poured a cup, the steam rising into the cool air of the tent.

"How was sick call?" I asked.

He took a sip of coffee.

"My God, that is good. The usual, colds, coughs, two cases of trench foot."

"Nothing serious?"

"Nothing needing a trip to the rear," Rossi replied.

"You know, as this bloody war winds down, there will be a great effort to not be the last man killed in the war."

"Do you blame them?" he asked.

"God no, I think we all feel the same way. But how do you get men to attack the enemy, knowing the end is in sight?"

"I'll leave that up to the colonel," Glen replied and poured more coffee into his cup.

"The word from the French troops is that the Kaiser has abdicated, surely that must mean the war will end."

Glen laughed.

"The rumor from division is that the war won't end until we have occupied Berlin."

Cold air entered as the tent flap was pushed aside. Rand entered.

"Good morning, all. I come bearing a message from our Executive Officer. He requests your attendance at a meeting of all senior officers."

"What time?"

"In twenty minutes, his tent."

"Thanks, Rand. Have some coffee while it's hot."

Lieutenant Colonel Abner Prescott sat at the small table at the end of his tent. Several officers sat in the three available chairs, while the rest of us stood behind them. A map lay on the table, which everyone could see.

"Here is our estimate of the position of the German infantry which appears to be in brigade strength. Aerial reconnaissance has seen a single battery of three field guns, but nothing else. The Third Division will be moving forward tomorrow to capture the main German railhead in the area. Our job is the protect their left flank from any interference from the German brigade. Our plan is to move out in company order, taking positions as noted on the map. Each company will take up blocking positions to prevent any attacks across this valley. Any questions so far?"

"How wide will our front be, sir?" Herb Turley asked.

"You've hit the key point. Our responsibility is for a defensive line almost two miles long. The obvious problem is that is too much territory for a battalion, much less an understrength battalion. But it is what it is. Our division is augmenting us with a machine gun company from the Royal Fusiliers. We'll set machine guns up in the gaps between our company areas. It's not a perfect solution, but it will prevent the Germans from easily attacking the 3rd Division's flank."

I am a doctor, not skilled in the art of war, but having been in this business for some time, it was clear we were going to be in a perilous position. If the German brigade chose to attack aggressively, we would be significantly outnumbered. My problem would be the furthest troops on the end of the line would be two miles from medical help. This was going to be a challenge.

The colonel went on to give us the timetable and specific codes and signals of the day.

He finished by addressing what was the highest on our minds.

"I know rumors are rampant. The Kaiser is out, peace has been signed, we will march to Berlin or home by Christmas. None of that is true as far as I know. What I do know is that we must keep our men focused. That is the way we will minimize casualties. That is your job, gentlemen. Make it so."

When the company officers broke to discuss their own issues, I left to convene our group.

Our own tactics and procedures had changed over the last six months. Having left the established trenches where we could build semi-permanent aid stations, we had adopted a tactic much like I first saw when I got to France. The aid station is really just a location with a doctor, one or two orderlies, and several teams of stretcher bearers. This time I think we need to change that up to deal with the large distances the teams would have to carry the wounded.

I had the entire medical staff together to go over the plan. The farthest aid station would be taken by Rand. I would take the next closest and Glen the station closest to the rear. We would have ten bearer teams. Five would start with Rand, three with me and two with Glen. Teams from Rand's air station would hand off their patient much like in a relay race, returning with their stretcher to their original station. If we had too many wounded, we would downsize the teams to two men each or commandeer local troops to help. We would count on having ambulances at the end of our evacuation line, and hope the German artillery did not have spotters.

"What time?" Glen asked.

"Sunrise, about 7:30. Which means we need to be ready to move out behind the lads right after that."

They nodded.

"Let's make sure we have our supplies ready and brief the stretcher teams. We'll have a busy afternoon."

The cold wind was accentuated as the sun went down. But our teams were ready. I recalled the phrase 'one more time into the breach.' What a play Mr. Shakespeare could write about this war.

Glen opened the flap and grinned.

"I come bearing gifts."

He carried a canvass bag, which he carefully placed on the small box we used for a table.

"Feast your eyes on this. From glorious Canada."

He held up a can of Canadian salmon. My God, that's like gold.

"Three cans from home, with canned pineapple for dessert."

I held up the salmon can, examining it in the lantern light. What a surprise.

"You, Lieutenant Rossi, have outdone yourself."

"Ah, but wait, we're not done.

He pulled a tin of Carr's Table Water Biscuits from his bag.

"Only the best in crackers for the best in salmon."

"My God, where did you get these?"

"From a friend who has access to supplies normally kept for the generals."

"I think this feast calls for my final bottle of Haig and Haig."

"And I will go find Doctor Bernard, who surely will enjoy our little party."

"At least we aren't going into battle with an empty stomach," Glen said, as he drank the last of the juice from a pineapple can."

"Thanks to you, my friend."

Rand raised his glass, then took a drink.

"Let's not do anything heroic tomorrow, gentlemen. The war may not be over, but it's damned close."

"Don't worry about this Canadian, my goal in life is to see the Pacific Ocean, from the western shore of Canada."

"I just want to see my wife, on whatever shore I might find her," Rand added.

I thought of Kathleen, the love I thought I would never find. Yes, I wanted to see her, every day for the rest of my life."

I raised my glass.

"I would raise my glass to you two. I could have not asked for better friends and colleagues."

We all drank and I thought of James. It seemed so long ago, but the loss never goes away.

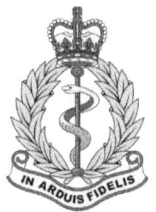

Chapter Forty-Four

"It was a little thing, but it was a victory."

Highland Light Infantry
Mons, Belgium
8 November 1918

As we were a blocking force, our advance was not preceded by an artillery barrage. The battalion line of advance was well clear of the German's machine gun range. The only danger was if the enemy brigade opened up with their field guns.

I sensed a resignation among the men as they moved out. There was little to no talking, not because it was prohibited, but the men had nothing to say. I felt the same way. Get this over with and God let our men survive.

The medical department stayed together until we dropped off Glen with his orderly, Corporal Stanton. The rest of us kept up with the second company until they stopped to dig in. Bill Bance and I turned to move 100 yards behind the company and set up our gear. Now we wait.

The division attack was very evident from the artillery and explosions. But our Germans were quiet. Would that they remain so.

Thirty minutes later, the first artillery fire was heard to our front, followed by the impact left of our position, but behind the company line. I was glad we had found a sheltered spot for our aid station and the three of us crouched down, helmets on and waited.

Suddenly an explosion erupted close by on our left, the whir and buzz of fragments whipping across our position, several tearing up the dirt. A brutal reminder of how dangerous artillery is to men in the open.

The ongoing barrage continued, but as of now, there had been no troop movement from the Germans. If they came at us, they would be greeted by our machine guns. God knows we had suffered from theirs too many times.

A stretcher team came across the field, carrying a wounded man.

"Over here," Bill Nance roared over the sound of the ongoing artillery fire.

The bearers reached us, lowering the stretcher.

"Shrapnel wound in the back," the leader said. "We used bandages, but no morphine."

While I didn't know the names of all of the battalion soldiers, I did know many.

"Private Beeman right?"

He nodded.

"Andy," he said, his face in a grimace.

"I need to look at your back, Andy, then, expect some morphine for the pain. Now, let's get you on your stomach."

Blood had soaked through the compress bandages, his shirt and tunic. The wound was large and the potential for internal injuries was high.

Removing the bloody bandage, I saw the shrapnel had torn across his back like a plowshare. Was there damage to his spine? I used a compress to remove the blood which continued to seep from the wound.

"Andy, can you move your feet for me?"

Both feet moved like little steps.

"Outstanding, very well done. Corporal, we need to flush the wound with Dakin's hypochlorite."

After flushing it was clear to me that the ribs had protected the critical internal organs. This was an ugly, painful, but not dangerous wound.

"Andy, we're going to turn you on your stomach."

Once on his stomach, I administered morphine, confident there were no complicating issues.

"Now, we are going to sit you up while we bandage your back. Then the lads will get you back to the ambulances. They will take you to the CCS. You are going to be fine, Andy.

As they carried him toward Glen's aid station, I felt good. One wound, not life threatening and one more lad safe to go home for good.

Exploding artillery shells began to hammer the German lines. About time for counter-battery fire. I knew the Royal Air Force had started using radios to spot for artillery batteries. Perhaps they would be able to pinpoint the German guns.

Another stretcher team approached us from the direction of Rand's aid station. There were five men carrying the casualty, odd certainly.

Another German artillery shell exploded, causing the team to lower the stretcher and lay flat. Shrapnel was a fickle weapon, sometimes all the damage went to one side, other times the killing zone was perfectly circular. Every time it made good sense to take cover.

The got back to their feet and made their way toward us allowing me to see that one of the men was leaning over the patient.

"It's the doc," the stretcher lead called as the crested a small hillock and brought the patient in.

Corporal Dwyer was holding a compress to Rand's neck, the blood loss was significant.

"Shrapnel, neck wound, bad bleeder, doc."

"Let me see," I said, kneeling down over Rand.

He was pale, but his eyes were open.

I saw what I feared and the blood told the story. The external jugular appeared to be damaged. If it was severed, Rand was dead, there was no way to save him.

"Down here, quick as you can."

The corporal knelt as the stretcher was lowered to the ground.

"Let me see.

Dwyer moved the bandage and blood swelled from the wound and down Rand's neck.

"Pressure back, hard!"

I turned to Nance.

"Bill, I need a surgical kit. Number one silk on a number two needle.

"Right."

If I could close off the vein, top and bottom and stop the blood loss, he would have a chance. God guide my hands.

"Corporal, when I tell you to pull the bandage, I need you to put hard pressure with you finger one inch above the wound. Bill, you do the same below. Understand?"

"Aye, sir," Dwyer chipped back.

"Ready," Bill said, handing me the needle.

"Have the Dakin's ready to wash the blood away."

"Right."

"Corporal, release the bandage and apply your pressure. Bill, flush the wound."

I saw the upper area in the wound was bleeding more that the lower. A quick set of stiches, with a reef knot, followed by the same on the lower wound."

"Flush!"

The bleeding had slowed, but not stopped. The blood made it difficult to get purchase. Another set of stiches, this time with a surgeon's knot put a solid block on the vein. The same below and one more flush showed the bleeding finally stopped.

"Ringer's"

"Right," Nance said and pulled a bottle from the haversack.

Leaning over Rand I saw his eyes open slightly.

"Still with us?"

A slight smile.

"Any Haig handy."

I realized my eyes were tearing up. Good Lord, what's wrong with me.

Taking Rand's hand, I held it tight.

"Yes, my friend."

Two men of the Second Battalion of the Highland Light Infantry died that day. Private Dorsey had only been with the battalion for less than a month, I don't think I ever met him. Corporal Mike Carpenter had been with the battalion for over three years. I knew him, not well, but enough to greet him in camp. I could only thank the Lord that the German commander decided to stay in their positions and not attack. You have to be thankful for the little things.

As we carried Rand back to the ambulance pick up point, I felt good. One man, one doctor would live to help the world heal from this monstrous assault on humanity. It was a little thing, but it was a victory.

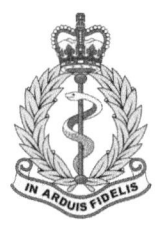

Epilogue

The end of hostilities came via the normal telegraph system:

```
Hostilities will cease 11.00 hours today
November 11.  Troops will stand fast at line
reached at that hour which will be reported by
wire to Corps headquarters.  Defensive
precautions will be maintained.  There will be
no intercourse of any description with the
enemy.
```

Once the relief reached everyone, the real question was when could we go home? In fact, the Highland Light Infantry was assigned to what came to be known as the "Army of the Rhine." We were going to move into Germany as part of the occupying forces. After spending four years on French territory, we crossed into Germany on the 9th of December, 1918. By Christmas, we were in place on the eastern side of Düren. We had no interaction with the German Army, all units having withdrawn over the Rhine in accordance with the armistice.

Kathleen remained at Boulogne as the hospital continued to care for the wounded from the last several months of fighting. She was finally sent home in April of 1919 as the hospital ceased operations. She remained with the Red Cross, taking up a nursing assignment at Springburn Hospital in Glasgow, which treated many returning servicemen.

Jonesy was demobilized when the hospital closed and traveled to Glasgow where he began assisting my father in his practice. Dan Jennings was sent to Erskine Hospital near Glasgow to have a prostheses manufactured and receive rehabilitation using the new leg.

The luck of having Kathleen, Ryan and Dan in Glasgow made every day for me in Germany bearable. It was strange we never knew what we were really supposed to be doing. There was no need for military force, the German police maintained order. We spent our time catching up on reading, writing letters and trying to accustom ourselves to life without a war. Finally in April of 1919, the battalion returned to Aldershot. I left active service at that time and returned to Glasgow. My war was finally over.

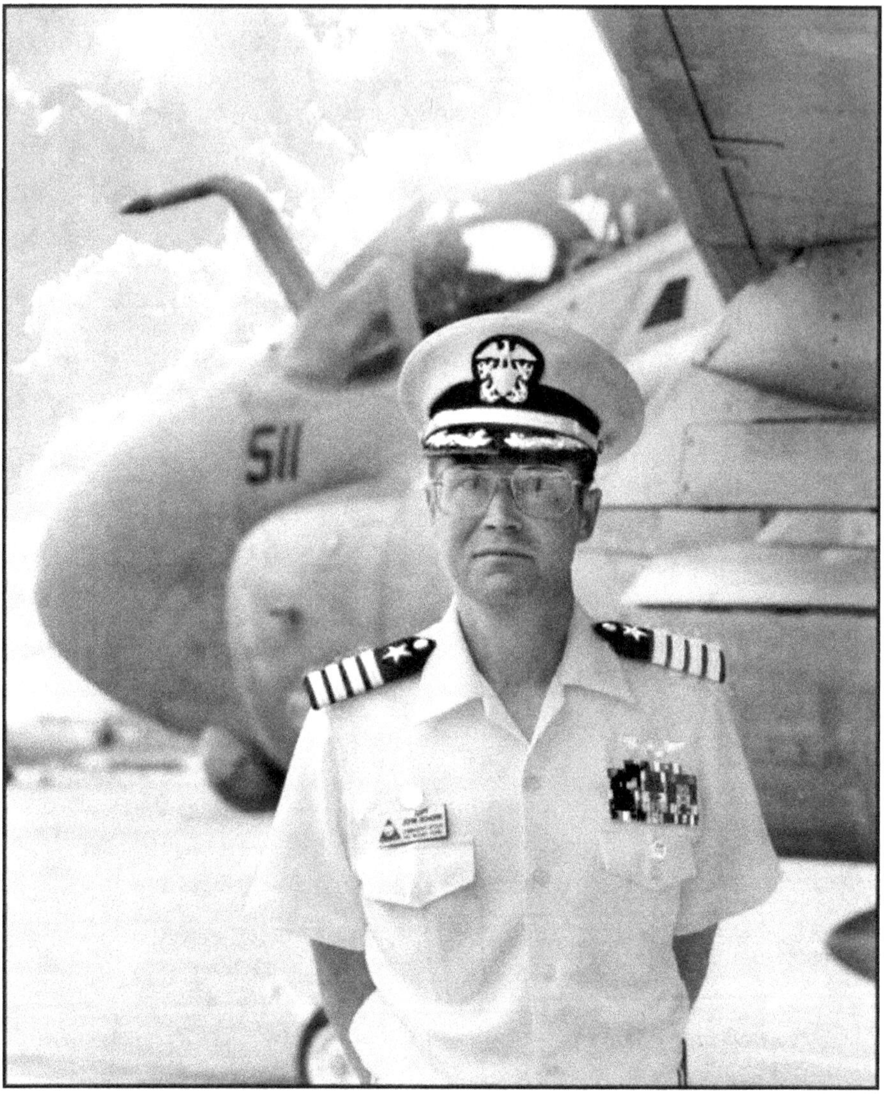

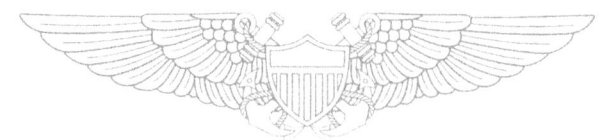

Captain John F. Schork
United States Navy, Ret.

ABOUT THE AUTHOR

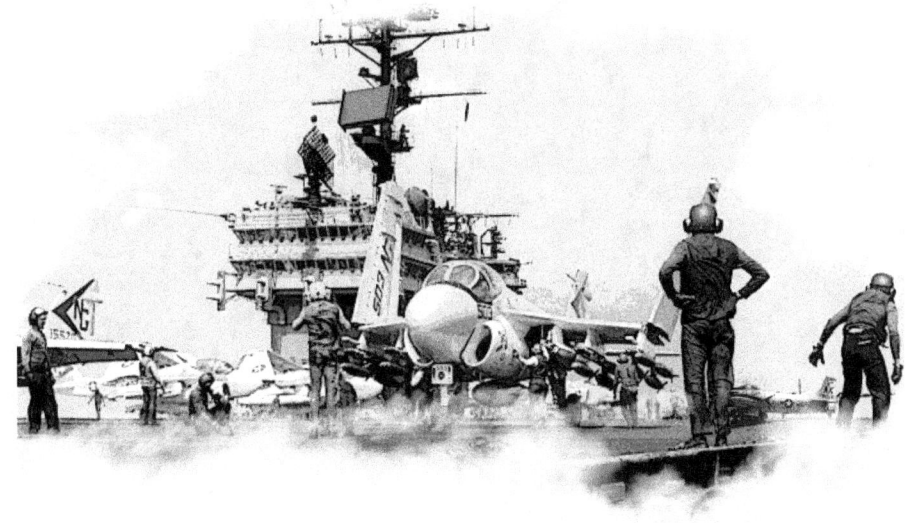

John Schork graduated from the U.S. Naval Academy in 1972 and went on to spend 26 years in Naval Aviation, flying the iconic Grumman A-6 Intruder.

During his career, he accumulated 4,000 flight hours and over 1,000 carrier arrested landings. Operating primarily in the Pacific theater, he took part in Operations Frequent Wind, Praying Mantis and Southern Watch among others.

As the last Executive Officer of the USS Midway (CV-41), he took part in Desert Storm and the evacuation of U.S. personnel from the Philippines following the eruption of Mt. Pinatubo. He commanded an A-6 Intruder Squadron, VA-95 and Naval Air Station Whidbey Island. His final tour was as the Chief of Staff of the Kitty Hawk Battle Group.

John is the author of adventure novels based upon historical events. He resides with his wife, Carole, in Sammamish, Washington.